DSM-5-TR®
Classification

DSM-5-TR®
Classification

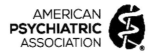

AMERICAN
PSYCHIATRIC
ASSOCIATION

Correspondence regarding copyright permissions should be directed to DSM Permissions, American Psychiatric Association Publishing, 800 Maine Ave. SW, Suite 900, Washington, DC 20024-2812.

If you wish to buy 50 or more copies of the same title, please go to www.appi.org/specialdiscounts for more information.

Manufactured in the United States of America on acid-free paper.
26 25 24   6 5
ISBN 978-0-89042-583-1 Fifth Printing, March 2024

American Psychiatric Association Publishing
800 Maine Avenue SW
Suite 900
Washington, DC 20024-2812
www.psychiatry.org

Contents

Introduction

The *DSM-5-TR Classification* provides readers with the DSM-5-TR classification of disorders and their identifying diagnostic and statistical ICD-10-CM codes presented in a handy format. First, the DSM-5-TR classification of disorders presents the diagnostic classes of disorders in the same sequence as in DSM-5-TR, beginning with Neurodevelopmental Disorders and ending with Other Mental Disorders. Within each diagnostic class, the specific disorders are also listed in the same sequence as they appear in DSM-5-TR. (As in DSM-5-TR, the classification also includes Medication-Induced Movement Disorders and Other Adverse Effects of Medication, as well as Other Conditions That May Be a Focus of Clinical Attention; these are not mental disorders but are conditions and problems that may be encountered by mental health clinicians). Next, the book contains an alphabetical listing of DSM-5 diagnoses with their associated ICD-10-CM codes. After the alphabetical listing, a numerical listing follows, with the ICD-10-CM codes for the DSM-5 diagnoses. The new DSM-5-TR disorder, prolonged grief disorder, is also included in the DSM-5-TR classification and code listings.

This book may be helpful for several types of readers, such as clinicians within a variety of disciplines, including psychiatrists, primary care physicians, psychologists, social workers, marriage and family therapists, and others who are providing clinical services to individuals with a mental disorder. It may serve as a useful resource for coders who work in medical centers and clinics and who are responsible for providing the proper diagnostic codes for the disorders that are a focus of clinical attention. It may also be a quick reference for insurance companies, which require that the proper diagnostic codes be used in order to determine whether the individual receiving clinical care is entitled to reimbursement for the condition being treated. Also, individuals conducting utilization or quality assurance reviews of specific cases will find this book useful. Finally, community mental health organizations at the state or county level may limit their services to individuals who have specific mental disorders, such as schizophrenia—and exclude other diagnoses, such as personality disorders. Consequently, each code and the associated disorder have important administrative implications.

For future periodic DSM-5-TR coding and other updates, see www.dsm5.org.

Coding and Recording Procedures

The official coding system in use in the United States since October 1, 2015, is the *International Classification of Diseases*, Tenth Revision, Clinical Modification (ICD-10-CM), a version of the World Health Organization's ICD-10 that has been modified for clinical use by the Centers for Disease Control and Prevention's National Center for Health Statistics (NCHS) and provides the only permissible diagnostic codes for mental disorders for clinical use in the United States. Most DSM-5 disorders have an alphanumeric ICD-10-CM code that appears preceding the name of the disorder (or coded subtype or specifier) in the DSM-5-TR Classification and in the accompanying criteria set for each disorder. For some diagnoses (e.g., neurocognitive disorders, substance/medication-induced disorders), the appropriate code depends on further specification and is listed within the criteria set for the disorder with a coding note, and in some cases is further clarified in the text section "Recording Procedures" in DSM-5-TR or the *Desk Reference to the Diagnostic Criteria From DSM-5-TR*. The names of some disorders are followed by alternative terms enclosed in parentheses.

The use of diagnostic codes is fundamental to medical record keeping. Diagnostic coding facilitates data collection and retrieval and compilation of statistical information. Codes also are often required to report diagnostic data to interested third parties, including governmental agencies, private insurers, and the World Health Organization. For example, in the United States, the use of ICD-10-CM codes for disorders in DSM-5-TR has been mandated by the Health Care Financing Administration for purposes of reimbursement under the Medicare system.

Principal Diagnosis/Reason for Visit

The general convention in DSM-5 is to allow multiple diagnoses to be assigned for those presentations that meet criteria for more than one DSM-5 disorder. When more than one diagnosis is given in an inpatient setting, the principal diagnosis is the condition established after study to be chiefly responsible for occasioning the admission of the individual. When more than one diagnosis is given for an individual in an outpatient setting, the reason for visit is the condition that is chiefly responsible for the ambulatory medical services received during the visit. In most cases, the principal diagnosis or the reason for visit is also the main focus of attention or treatment. It is often difficult (and somewhat arbitrary) to determine which diagnosis is the principal diagnosis or the reason for visit. For example, it may be unclear which diagnosis should be considered "principal" for an individual hospitalized with both schizophrenia and alcohol use disorder, because each condition may have contributed equally to the need for admission and treatment.

The principal diagnosis is indicated by listing it first, and the remaining disorders are listed in order of focus of attention and treatment. When the principal diagnosis or reason for visit is a mental disorder due to another medical condition (e.g., major neurocognitive disorder due to Alzheimer's disease, psychotic disorder due to malignant lung neoplasm), ICD coding rules require that the etiological medical condition be listed first. In that case, the principal diagnosis or reason for visit would be the mental disorder due to the medical condition, the second listed diagnosis. For maximum clarity, the disorder listed as the principal diagnosis or the reason for visit can be followed by the qualifying phrase "(principal diagnosis)" or "(reason for visit)."

Provisional Diagnosis

The modifier "provisional" can be used when there is currently insufficient information to indicate that the diagnostic criteria are met, but there is a strong presumption that the information will become available to allow that determination. The clinician can indicate the diagnostic uncertainty by recording "(provisional)" following the diagnosis. For example, this modifier might be used when an individual who appears to have a presentation consistent with a diagnosis of current major depressive disorder is unable to give an adequate history, but it is expected that such information will become available after interviewing an informant or reviewing medical records. Once that information becomes available and confirms that the diagnostic criteria were met, the modifier "(provisional)" would be removed. Another use of "provisional" is for those situations in which differential diagnosis depends exclusively on whether the duration of illness does not exceed an upper limit as required by the diagnostic criteria. For example, a diagnosis of schizophreniform disorder requires a duration of at least 1 month but less than 6 months. If an individual currently has symptoms consistent with a diagnosis of schizophreniform disorder except that the ultimate duration is unknown because the symptoms are still ongoing, the modifier "(provisional)" would be applied and then removed if the symptoms remit within a period of 6 months. If they do not remit, the diagnosis would be changed to schizophrenia.

Subtypes and Specifiers

Subtypes and specifiers are provided for increased diagnostic specificity. Subtypes define mutually exclusive and jointly exhaustive phenomenological subgroupings within a diagnosis and are indicated by the instruction "*Specify* whether" in the criteria set (e.g., in anorexia nervosa, *Specify* whether restricting type or binge-eating/purging type). In contrast, specifiers are not intended to be mutually exclusive or jointly exhaustive, and as a consequence, more than one specifier may be applied to a given diagnosis. Specifiers (as opposed to subtypes) are indicated by the instruction "*Specify*" or "*Specify* if" in the criteria set (e.g., in social anxiety disorder, "*Specify* if: performance only"). Specifiers and subtypes provide an opportunity to define a more homogeneous subgrouping of individuals with the disorder who share certain features (e.g., major depressive disorder, with mixed features) and to convey information that is relevant to the management of the individual's disorder, such as the "with other medical comorbidity" specifier in sleep-wake disorders. Although the fifth character within an ICD-10-CM code is sometimes designated to indicate a particular subtype or specifier (e.g., "0" in the fifth character in the F06.70 diagnostic code for mild neurocognitive disorder due to traumatic brain injury, to indicate the absence of a behavioral disturbance vs. a "1" in the fifth character of the F06.71 diagnostic code for mild neurocognitive disorder due to traumatic brain injury to indicate the presence of a behavioral disturbance), the majority of subtypes and specifiers included in DSM-5-TR are not reflected in the ICD-10-CM code and are indicated instead by recording the subtype or specifier after the name of the disorder (e.g., social anxiety disorder, performance type).

Substance/Medication-Induced Mental Disorders

The term *substance/medication-induced mental disorder* refers to symptomatic presentations that are due to the physiological effects of an exogenous substance on the central nervous system, including symptoms that develop during withdrawal from an exogenous substance that is capable of causing physiological dependence. Such exogenous substances include typical intoxicants (e.g., alcohol, inhalants, hallucinogens, cocaine), psychotropic medications (e.g., stimulants; sedatives, hypnotics, anxiolytics), other medications (e.g., steroids), and environmental toxins (e.g., organophosphate insecticides).

When recording the name of the disorder, the comorbid substance use disorder (if any) is listed first, followed by the word "with," followed by the name of the specific substance that induced the specific mental disorder, followed by the specification of onset (i.e., onset during intoxication, onset during withdrawal). See the section "Recording Procedures" for these diagnoses in DSM-5-TR or the *Desk Reference to the Diagnostic Criteria From DSM-5-TR* for further guidance.

Other Specified and Unspecified Mental Disorders

DSM-5 provides two diagnostic options for presentations that do not meet the diagnostic criteria for any of the specific DSM-5 disorders: other specified disorder and unspecified disorder. The other specified category is provided to allow the clinician to communicate the specific reason that the presentation does not meet the criteria for any specific category within a diagnostic class. This is done by recording the name of the category, followed by the specific reason. If the clinician chooses not to specify the reason that the criteria are not met for a specific disorder, then the unspecified category would be diagnosed. Note that the differentiation between other specified and unspecified disorders is based on the clinician's choice to indicate or not the reasons why the presentation does not meet full criteria, providing maximum flexibility for diagnosis. When the clinician determines that there is enough available clinical information to specify the nature of the presentation, the "other specified" diagnosis can be given. In those cases where the clinician is not able to further specify the clinical presentation (e.g., in emergency room settings), the "unspecified" diagnosis can be given. This is entirely a matter of clinical judgment. See

DSM-5-TR "Use of the Manual" for more information on these diagnoses.

Harmonization With ICD-11

Because of differences in timing, complete harmonization of the DSM-5 diagnostic criteria with the ICD-11 disorder definitions was not possible because the DSM-5 developmental effort was several years ahead of the ICD-11 revision process. Consequently, the DSM-5 diagnostic criteria were finalized just as the ICD-11 working groups were beginning to develop the ICD-11 clinical descriptions and diagnostic guidelines. Some improvement in harmonization at the disorder level was still achieved; many ICD-11 working group members had participated in the development of the DSM-5 diagnostic criteria, and the ICD-11 working groups were instructed to review the DSM-5 criteria sets and strive to make ICD-11 diagnostic guidelines as similar to DSM-5 as possible unless there was a considered reason for them to differ.

Although ICD-11 was officially endorsed for use by the World Health Organization member nations during the 72nd World Health Assembly in May 2019 and officially came into effect on January 1, 2022, each country chooses when to adopt ICD-11. There is currently no proposed timeline for implementation of ICD-11 in the United States. Consequently, for the foreseeable future the official coding system in the United States continues to be ICD-10-CM.

Cautionary Note

The DSM-5-TR Classification should not be used by clinicians on its own. This resource is primarily intended to be a readily accessible reference only to the ICD-10-CM codes for DSM-5 diagnoses. Clinicians are strongly encouraged to use this book as a companion to DSM-5-TR or the *Desk Reference to the Diagnostic Criteria From DSM-5-TR*, where the diagnostic criteria and other explanatory information are presented.

References

American Psychiatric Association: Diagnostic and Statistical Manual of Mental Disorders, 5th Edition, Text Revision. Washington, DC, American Psychiatric Association, 2022

American Psychiatric Association: Desk Reference to the Diagnostic Criteria From DSM-5-TR. Washington, DC, American Psychiatric Association, 2022

Before each disorder name, ICD-10-CM codes are provided. Blank lines indicate that the ICD-10-CM code depends on the applicable subtype, specifier, or class of substance. For periodic DSM-5-TR coding and other updates, see www.dsm5.org.

Following chapter titles and disorder names, page numbers for the corresponding text or criteria are included in parentheses.

Note for all mental disorders due to another medical condition: Insert the name of the etiological medical condition within the name of the mental disorder due to [the medical condition]. The code and name for the etiological medical condition should be listed first immediately before the mental disorder due to the medical condition.

Neurodevelopmental Disorders

Intellectual Developmental Disorders

___.___   Intellectual Developmental Disorder (Intellectual Disability)
         Specify current severity:

F70   Mild

F71   Moderate

F72   Severe

F73   Profound

F88   Global Developmental Delay

F79   Unspecified Intellectual Developmental Disorder (Intellectual Disability)

Communication Disorders

F80.2   Language Disorder

F80.0   Speech Sound Disorder

F80.81   Childhood-Onset Fluency Disorder (Stuttering)
             Note: Later-onset cases are diagnosed as F98.5 adult-onset flu-
             ency disorder.

F80.82   Social (Pragmatic) Communication Disorder

F80.9   Unspecified Communication Disorder

Autism Spectrum Disorder

F84.0   Autism Spectrum Disorder
             Specify current severity: Requiring very substantial support,
             Requiring substantial support, Requiring support
             Specify if: With or without accompanying intellectual impair-
             ment, With or without accompanying language impair-
             ment
             Specify if: Associated with a known genetic or other medical
             condition or environmental factor (**Coding note:** Use addi-
             tional code to identify the associated genetic or other med-
             ical condition); Associated with a neurodevelopmental,
             mental, or behavioral problem
             Specify if: With catatonia (use additional code F06.1)

Attention-Deficit/Hyperactivity Disorder

___.__   Attention-Deficit/Hyperactivity Disorder
             Specify if: In partial remission
             Specify current severity: Mild, Moderate, Severe
             Specify whether:

F90.2   Combined presentation

F90.0   Predominantly inattentive presentation

F90.1   Predominantly hyperactive/impulsive presentation

F90.8   Other Specified Attention-Deficit/Hyperactivity Disorder

F90.9   Unspecified Attention-Deficit/Hyperactivity Disorder

Specific Learning Disorder

___.__   Specific Learning Disorder
             Specify current severity: Mild, Moderate, Severe

Specify if:

F81.0	With impairment in reading (specify if with word reading accuracy, reading rate or fluency, reading comprehension)
F81.81	With impairment in written expression (specify if with spelling accuracy, grammar and punctuation accuracy, clarity or organization of written expression)
F81.2	With impairment in mathematics (specify if with number sense, memorization of arithmetic facts, accurate or fluent calculation, accurate math reasoning)

Motor Disorders

F82 Developmental Coordination Disorder

F98.4 Stereotypic Movement Disorder
Specify if: With self-injurious behavior, Without self-injurious behavior
Specify if: Associated with a known genetic or other medical condition, neurodevelopmental disorder, or environmental factor
Specify current severity: Mild, Moderate, Severe

Tic Disorders

F95.2 Tourette's Disorder

F95.1 Persistent (Chronic) Motor or Vocal Tic Disorder
Specify if: With motor tics only, With vocal tics only

F95.0 Provisional Tic Disorder

F95.8 Other Specified Tic Disorder

F95.9 Unspecified Tic Disorder

Other Neurodevelopmental Disorders

F88 Other Specified Neurodevelopmental Disorder

F89 Unspecified Neurodevelopmental Disorder

Schizophrenia Spectrum and Other Psychotic Disorders

The following specifiers apply to Schizophrenia Spectrum and Other Psychotic Disorders where indicated:

[a]*Specify* if: The following course specifiers are only to be used after a 1-year duration of the disorder: First episode, currently in acute episode; First episode, currently in partial remission; First episode, currently in full remission; Multiple episodes, currently in acute episode; Multiple episodes, currently in partial remission; Multiple episodes, currently in full remission; Continuous; Unspecified

[b]*Specify* if: With catatonia (use additional code F06.1)

[c]*Specify* current severity of delusions, hallucinations, disorganized speech, abnormal psychomotor behavior, negative symptoms, impaired cognition, depression, and mania symptoms

F21	Schizotypal (Personality) Disorder
F22	Delusional Disorder[a,c]

      Specify whether: Erotomanic type, Grandiose type, Jealous type, Persecutory type, Somatic type, Mixed type, Unspecified type

      Specify if: With bizarre content

F23	Brief Psychotic Disorder[b,c]

      Specify if: With marked stressor(s), Without marked stressor(s), With peripartum onset

F20.81	Schizophreniform Disorder[b,c]

      Specify if: With good prognostic features, Without good prognostic features

F20.9	Schizophrenia[a,b,c]
___.__	Schizoaffective Disorder[a,b,c]

      Specify whether:

F25.0	Bipolar type
F25.1	Depressive type
___.__	Substance/Medication-Induced Psychotic Disorder[c]

      Note: For applicable ICD-10-CM codes, refer to the substance classes under Substance-Related and Addictive Disorders for the specific substance/medication-induced psychotic

disorder. See also the criteria set and corresponding recording procedures in the manual for more information.

Coding note: The ICD-10-CM code depends on whether or not
there is a comorbid substance use disorder present for the
same class of substance. In any case, an additional separate
diagnosis of a substance use disorder is not given.

Specify if: With onset during intoxication, With onset during
withdrawal, With onset after medication use

___.__	Psychotic Disorder Due to Another Medical Condition[c]

Specify whether:

F06.2	With delusions
F06.0	With hallucinations
F06.1	Catatonia Associated With Another Mental Disorder (Catatonia Specifier)
F06.1	Catatonic Disorder Due to Another Medical Condition
F06.1	Unspecified Catatonia

Note: Code first **R29.818** other symptoms involving nervous
and musculoskeletal systems.

F28	Other Specified Schizophrenia Spectrum and Other Psychotic Disorder
F29	Unspecified Schizophrenia Spectrum and Other Psychotic Disorder

---

Bipolar and Related Disorders

The following specifiers apply to Bipolar and Related Disorders where indicated:

[a]*Specify:* With anxious distress (*specify* current severity: mild, moderate,
moderate-severe, severe); With mixed features; With rapid cycling;
With melancholic features; With atypical features; With mood-congru-
ent psychotic features; With mood-incongruent psychotic features;
With catatonia (use additional code F06.1); With peripartum onset;
With seasonal pattern

[b]*Specify:* With anxious distress (*specify* current severity: mild, moderate,
moderate-severe, severe); With mixed features; With rapid cycling; With
peripartum onset; With seasonal pattern

___.__ Bipolar I Disorder[a]

___.__   Current or most recent episode manic

F31.11   Mild

F31.12   Moderate

F31.13   Severe

F31.2   With psychotic features

F31.73   In partial remission

F31.74   In full remission

F31.9   Unspecified

F31.0   Current or most recent episode hypomanic

F31.71   In partial remission

F31.72   In full remission

F31.9   Unspecified

___.__   Current or most recent episode depressed

F31.31   Mild

F31.32   Moderate

F31.4   Severe

F31.5   With psychotic features

F31.75   In partial remission

F31.76   In full remission

F31.9   Unspecified

F31.9   Current or most recent episode unspecified

F31.81 Bipolar II Disorder

Specify current or most recent episode: Hypomanic[b], Depressed[a]

Specify course if full criteria for a mood episode are not currently met: In partial remission, In full remission

Specify severity if full criteria for a major depressive episode are currently met: Mild, Moderate, Severe

F34.0 Cyclothymic Disorder

Specify if: With anxious distress (*specify* current severity: mild, moderate, moderate-severe, severe)

___.__ Substance/Medication-Induced Bipolar and Related Disorder

Note: For applicable ICD-10-CM codes, refer to the substance classes under Substance-Related and Addictive Disorders for the specific substance/medication-induced bipolar and related disorder. See also the criteria set and corresponding recording procedures in the manual for more information.

> **Coding note:** The ICD-10-CM code depends on whether or not there is a comorbid substance use disorder present for the same class of substance. In any case, an additional separate diagnosis of a substance use disorder is not given.
> *Specify* if: With onset during intoxication, With onset during withdrawal, With onset after medication use

___.___ Bipolar and Related Disorder Due to Another Medical Condition
> *Specify* if:

F06.33 With manic features

F06.33 With manic- or hypomanic-like episode

F06.34 With mixed features

F31.89 Other Specified Bipolar and Related Disorder

F31.9 Unspecified Bipolar and Related Disorder

F39 Unspecified Mood Disorder

Depressive Disorders

F34.81 Disruptive Mood Dysregulation Disorder

___.___ Major Depressive Disorder
> *Specify:* With anxious distress (*specify* current severity: mild, moderate, moderate-severe, severe); With mixed features; With melancholic features; With atypical features; With mood-congruent psychotic features; With mood-incongruent psychotic features; With catatonia (use additional code F06.1); With peripartum onset; With seasonal pattern

___.___ Single episode

F32.0 Mild

F32.1 Moderate

F32.2 Severe

F32.3 With psychotic features

F32.4 In partial remission

F32.5 In full remission

F32.9 Unspecified

___.___ Recurrent episode

F33.0 Mild

F33.1 Moderate

F33.2   Severe
F33.3   With psychotic features
F33.41   In partial remission
F33.42   In full remission
F33.9   Unspecified

F34.1   Persistent Depressive Disorder
                   Specify: With anxious distress (*specify* current severity: mild,
                        moderate, moderate-severe, severe); With atypical fea-
                        tures
                   Specify if: In partial remission, In full remission
                   Specify if: Early onset, Late onset
                   Specify if: With pure dysthymic syndrome; With persistent ma-
                        jor depressive episode; With intermittent major depressive
                        episodes, with current episode; With intermittent major
                        depressive episodes, without current episode
                   Specify current severity: Mild, Moderate, Severe

F32.81   Premenstrual Dysphoric Disorder

___.___   Substance/Medication-Induced Depressive Disorder
                   Note: For applicable ICD-10-CM codes, refer to the substance
                        classes under Substance-Related and Addictive Disorders
                        for the specific substance/medication-induced depressive
                        disorder. See also the criteria set and corresponding re-
                        cording procedures in the manual for more information.
                   Coding note: The ICD-10-CM code depends on whether or not
                        there is a comorbid substance use disorder present for the
                        same class of substance. In any case, an additional separate
                        diagnosis of a substance use disorder is not given.
                   Specify if: With onset during intoxication, With onset during
                        withdrawal, With onset after medication use

___.___   Depressive Disorder Due to Another Medical Condition
                   Specify if:
F06.31   With depressive features
F06.32   With major depressive–like episode
F06.34   With mixed features

F32.89   Other Specified Depressive Disorder

F32.A   Unspecified Depressive Disorder

F39   Unspecified Mood Disorder

Anxiety Disorders

F93.0   Separation Anxiety Disorder

F94.0   Selective Mutism

___.___   Specific Phobia
            Specify if:
F40.218   Animal
F40.228   Natural environment
___.___   Blood-injection-injury
F40.230   Fear of blood
F40.231   Fear of injections and transfusions
F40.232   Fear of other medical care
F40.233   Fear of injury
F40.248   Situational
F40.298   Other

F40.10   Social Anxiety Disorder
            Specify if: Performance only

F41.0   Panic Disorder

___.___   Panic Attack Specifier

F40.00   Agoraphobia

F41.1   Generalized Anxiety Disorder

___.___   Substance/Medication-Induced Anxiety Disorder
            Note: For applicable ICD-10-CM codes, refer to the substance
                classes under Substance-Related and Addictive Disorders
                for the specific substance/medication-induced anxiety
                disorder. See also the criteria set and corresponding re-
                cording procedures in the manual for more information.
            Coding note: The ICD-10-CM code depends on whether or not
                there is a comorbid substance use disorder present for the
                same class of substance. In any case, an additional separate
                diagnosis of a substance use disorder is not given.
            Specify if: With onset during intoxication, With onset during
                withdrawal, With onset after medication use

F06.4   Anxiety Disorder Due to Another Medical Condition

F41.8   Other Specified Anxiety Disorder

F41.9   Unspecified Anxiety Disorder

Obsessive-Compulsive and Related Disorders

The following specifier applies to Obsessive-Compulsive and Related Disorders where indicated:

[a]*Specify* if: With good or fair insight, With poor insight, With absent insight/delusional beliefs

F42.2   Obsessive-Compulsive Disorder[a]
            Specify if: Tic-related

F45.22 Body Dysmorphic Disorder[a]
            Specify if: With muscle dysmorphia

F42.3   Hoarding Disorder[a]
            Specify if: With excessive acquisition

F63.3   Trichotillomania (Hair-Pulling Disorder)

F42.4   Excoriation (Skin-Picking) Disorder

___.__ Substance/Medication-Induced Obsessive-Compulsive and Related Disorder
            Note: For applicable ICD-10-CM codes, refer to the substance classes under Substance-Related and Addictive Disorders for the specific substance/medication-induced obsessive-compulsive and related disorder. See also the criteria set and corresponding recording procedures in the manual for more information.
            Coding note: The ICD-10-CM code depends on whether or not there is a comorbid substance use disorder present for the same class of substance. In any case, an additional separate diagnosis of a substance use disorder is not given.
            Specify if: With onset during intoxication, With onset during withdrawal, With onset after medication use

F06.8   Obsessive-Compulsive and Related Disorder Due to Another Medical Condition
            Specify if: With obsessive-compulsive disorder–like symptoms, With appearance preoccupations, With hoarding symptoms, With hair-pulling symptoms, With skin-picking symptoms

F42.8   Other Specified Obsessive-Compulsive and Related
             Disorder

F42.9   Unspecified Obsessive-Compulsive and Related Disorder

---

Trauma- and Stressor-Related Disorders

F94.1   Reactive Attachment Disorder
             Specify if: Persistent
             Specify current severity: Severe

F94.2   Disinhibited Social Engagement Disorder
             Specify if: Persistent
             Specify current severity: Severe

F43.10 Posttraumatic Stress Disorder
             Specify whether: With dissociative symptoms
             Specify if: With delayed expression

___.___   Posttraumatic Stress Disorder in Individuals Older
             Than 6 Years

___.___   Posttraumatic Stress Disorder in Children 6 Years and
             Younger

F43.0   Acute Stress Disorder

___.___   Adjustment Disorders
             Specify if: Acute, Persistent (chronic)
             Specify whether:

F43.21   With depressed mood

F43.22   With anxiety

F43.23   With mixed anxiety and depressed mood

F43.24   With disturbance of conduct

F43.25   With mixed disturbance of emotions and conduct

F43.20   Unspecified

F43.81 Prolonged Grief Disorder

F43.89 Other Specified Trauma- and Stressor-Related Disorder

F43.9   Unspecified Trauma- and Stressor-Related Disorder

Dissociative Disorders

F44.81 Dissociative Identity Disorder

F44.0 Dissociative Amnesia
            Specify if:
F44.1   With dissociative fugue

F48.1 Depersonalization/Derealization Disorder

F44.89 Other Specified Dissociative Disorder

F44.9 Unspecified Dissociative Disorder

Somatic Symptom and Related Disorders

F45.1 Somatic Symptom Disorder
            Specify if: With predominant pain
            Specify if: Persistent
            Specify current severity: Mild, Moderate, Severe

F45.21 Illness Anxiety Disorder
            Specify whether: Care-seeking type, Care-avoidant type

___.__ Functional Neurological Symptom Disorder (Conversion
            Disorder)
            Specify if: Acute episode, Persistent
            Specify if: With psychological stressor (specify stressor), With-
            out psychological stressor
            Specify symptom type:
F44.4   With weakness or paralysis
F44.4   With abnormal movement
F44.4   With swallowing symptoms
F44.4   With speech symptom
F44.5   With attacks or seizures
F44.6   With anesthesia or sensory loss
F44.6   With special sensory symptom
F44.7   With mixed symptoms

F54 Psychological Factors Affecting Other Medical Conditions
         Specify current severity: Mild, Moderate, Severe, Extreme

___.___   Factitious Disorder
         Specify: Single episode, Recurrent episodes
F68.10   Factitious Disorder Imposed on Self
F68.A   Factitious Disorder Imposed on Another
F45.8   Other Specified Somatic Symptom and Related Disorder
F45.9   Unspecified Somatic Symptom and Related Disorder

Feeding and Eating Disorders

The following specifiers apply to Feeding and Eating Disorders where indicated:
[a]*Specify* if: In remission
[b]*Specify* if: In partial remission, In full remission
[c]*Specify* current severity: Mild, Moderate, Severe, Extreme

___.___   Pica[a]
F98.3   In children
F50.89   In adults
F98.21   Rumination Disorder[a]
F50.82   Avoidant/Restrictive Food Intake Disorder[a]
___.___   Anorexia Nervosa[b,c]
         Specify whether:
F50.01   Restricting type
F50.02   Binge-eating/purging type
F50.2   Bulimia Nervosa[b,c]
F50.81   Binge-Eating Disorder[b,c]
F50.89   Other Specified Feeding or Eating Disorder
F50.9   Unspecified Feeding or Eating Disorder

Elimination Disorders

F98.0   Enuresis
         Specify whether: Nocturnal only, Diurnal only, Nocturnal and
         diurnal

F98.1   Encopresis
              Specify whether: With constipation and overflow incontinence,
                   Without constipation and overflow incontinence

___.___   Other Specified Elimination Disorder
N39.498   With urinary symptoms
R15.9   With fecal symptoms

___.___   Unspecified Elimination Disorder
R32   With urinary symptoms
R15.9   With fecal symptoms

Sleep-Wake Disorders

The following specifiers apply to Sleep-Wake Disorders where indicated:
[a]*Specify* if: Episodic, Persistent, Recurrent
[b]*Specify* if: Acute, Subacute, Persistent
[c]*Specify* current severity: Mild, Moderate, Severe

F51.01   Insomnia Disorder[a]
              Specify if: With mental disorder, With medical condition, With
                   another sleep disorder

F51.11   Hypersomnolence Disorder[b,c]
              Specify if: With mental disorder, With medical condition, With
                   another sleep disorder

___.___   Narcolepsy[c]
              Specify whether:
G47.411   Narcolepsy with cataplexy or hypocretin deficiency
                        (type 1)
G47.419   Narcolepsy without cataplexy and either without
                        hypocretin deficiency or hypocretin unmeasured
                        (type 2)
G47.421   Narcolepsy with cataplexy or hypocretin deficiency
                        due to a medical condition
G47.429   Narcolepsy without cataplexy and without hypocretin
                        deficiency due to a medical condition

Breathing-Related Sleep Disorders

G47.33 Obstructive Sleep Apnea Hypopnea[c]

___.___   Central Sleep Apnea
          Specify current severity
          Specify whether:
G47.31   Idiopathic central sleep apnea
R06.3   Cheyne-Stokes breathing
G47.37   Central sleep apnea comorbid with opioid use
               Note: First code opioid use disorder, if present.

___.___   Sleep-Related Hypoventilation
          Specify current severity
          Specify whether:
G47.34   Idiopathic hypoventilation
G47.35   Congenital central alveolar hypoventilation
G47.36   Comorbid sleep-related hypoventilation

___.___   Circadian Rhythm Sleep-Wake Disorders[a]
          Specify whether:
G47.21   Delayed sleep phase type
          Specify if: Familial, Overlapping with non-24-hour sleep-wake
               type
G47.22   Advanced sleep phase type
               Specify if: Familial
G47.23   Irregular sleep-wake type
G47.24   Non-24-hour sleep-wake type
G47.26   Shift work type
G47.20   Unspecified type

Parasomnias

__.___   Non–Rapid Eye Movement Sleep Arousal Disorders
          Specify whether:
F51.3   Sleepwalking type
          Specify if: With sleep-related eating, With sleep-related sexual
               behavior (sexsomnia)
F51.4   Sleep terror type

F51.5   Nightmare Disorder[b,c]
Specify if: During sleep onset
Specify if: With mental disorder, With medical condition, With another sleep disorder

G47.52   Rapid Eye Movement Sleep Behavior Disorder

G25.81   Restless Legs Syndrome

___.__   Substance/Medication-Induced Sleep Disorder
Note: For applicable ICD-10-CM codes, refer to the substance classes under Substance-Related and Addictive Disorders for the specific substance/medication-induced sleep disorder. See also the criteria set and corresponding recording procedures in the manual for more information.
Coding note: The ICD-10-CM code depends on whether or not there is a comorbid substance use disorder present for the same class of substance. In any case, an additional separate diagnosis of a substance use disorder is not given.
Specify whether: Insomnia type, Daytime sleepiness type, Parasomnia type, Mixed type
Specify if: With onset during intoxication, With onset during withdrawal, With onset after medication use

G47.09   Other Specified Insomnia Disorder

G47.00   Unspecified Insomnia Disorder

G47.19   Other Specified Hypersomnolence Disorder

G47.10   Unspecified Hypersomnolence Disorder

G47.8   Other Specified Sleep-Wake Disorder

G47.9   Unspecified Sleep-Wake Disorder

Sexual Dysfunctions

The following specifiers apply to Sexual Dysfunctions where indicated:
[a]Specify whether: Lifelong, Acquired
[b]Specify whether: Generalized, Situational
[c]Specify current severity: Mild, Moderate, Severe

F52.32   Delayed Ejaculation[a,b,c]

F52.21   Erectile Disorder[a,b,c]

F52.31 Female Orgasmic Disorder[a,b,c]
            Specify if: Never experienced an orgasm under any situation

F52.22 Female Sexual Interest/Arousal Disorder[a,b,c]

F52.6   Genito-Pelvic Pain/Penetration Disorder[a,c]

F52.0   Male Hypoactive Sexual Desire Disorder[a,b,c]

F52.4   Premature (Early) Ejaculation[a,b,c]

___.___ Substance/Medication-Induced Sexual Dysfunction[c]
            Note: For applicable ICD-10-CM codes, refer to the substance
            classes under Substance-Related and Addictive Disorders
            for the specific substance/medication-induced sexual dys-
            function. See also the criteria set and corresponding re-
            cording procedures in the manual for more information.
            Coding note: The ICD-10-CM code depends on whether or not
            there is a comorbid substance use disorder present for the
            same class of substance. In any case, an additional separate
            diagnosis of a substance use disorder is not given.
            Specify if: With onset during intoxication, With onset during
            withdrawal, With onset after medication use

F52.8   Other Specified Sexual Dysfunction

F52.9   Unspecified Sexual Dysfunction

Gender Dysphoria

The following specifier and note apply to Gender Dysphoria where indicated:
[a]*Specify* if: With a disorder/difference of sex development
[b]**Note:** Code the disorder/difference of sex development if present, in ad-
dition to gender dysphoria.

___.___ Gender Dysphoria

F64.2   Gender Dysphoria in Children[a,b]

F64.0   Gender Dysphoria in Adolescents and Adults[a,b]
            Specify if: Posttransition

F64.8   Other Specified Gender Dysphoria

F64.9   Unspecified Gender Dysphoria

Disruptive, Impulse-Control, and Conduct Disorders

F91.3   Oppositional Defiant Disorder
            Specify current severity: Mild, Moderate, Severe

F63.81 Intermittent Explosive Disorder

__.__   Conduct Disorder
            Specify if: With limited prosocial emotions
            Specify current severity: Mild, Moderate, Severe
            Specify whether:
F91.1   Childhood-onset type
F91.2   Adolescent-onset type
F91.9   Unspecified onset

F60.2   Antisocial Personality Disorder

F63.1   Pyromania

F63.2   Kleptomania

F91.8   Other Specified Disruptive, Impulse-Control, and
            Conduct Disorder

F91.9   Unspecified Disruptive, Impulse-Control, and Conduct
            Disorder

Substance-Related and Addictive Disorders

Substance-Related Disorders

Alcohol-Related Disorders

__.__   Alcohol Use Disorder
            Specify if: In a controlled environment
            Specify current severity/remission:
F10.10   Mild
F10.11   In early remission
F10.11   In sustained remission

F10.20	Moderate
F10.21	In early remission
F10.21	In sustained remission
F10.20	Severe
F10.21	In early remission
F10.21	In sustained remission
___.__	Alcohol Intoxication
F10.120	With mild use disorder
F10.220	With moderate or severe use disorder
F10.920	Without use disorder
___.__	Alcohol Withdrawal
	Without perceptual disturbances
F10.130	With mild use disorder
F10.230	With moderate or severe use disorder
F10.930	Without use disorder
	With perceptual disturbances
F10.132	With mild use disorder
F10.232	With moderate or severe use disorder
F10.932	Without use disorder
___.__	Alcohol-Induced Mental Disorders

___.__ Alcohol-Induced Mental Disorders
Note: Disorders are listed in their order of appearance in the manual.
[a]*Specify* With onset during intoxication, With onset during withdrawal
[b]*Specify* if: Acute, Persistent
[c]*Specify* if: Hyperactive, Hypoactive, Mixed level of activity

___.__	Alcohol-Induced Psychotic Disorder[a]
F10.159	With mild use disorder
F10.259	With moderate or severe use disorder
F10.959	Without use disorder
___.__	Alcohol-Induced Bipolar and Related Disorder[a]
F10.14	With mild use disorder
F10.24	With moderate or severe use disorder
F10.94	Without use disorder

___.__   Alcohol-Induced Depressive Disorder[a]
F10.14   With mild use disorder
F10.24   With moderate or severe use disorder
F10.94   Without use disorder

___.__   Alcohol-Induced Anxiety Disorder[a]
F10.180   With mild use disorder
F10.280   With moderate or severe use disorder
F10.980   Without use disorder

___.__   Alcohol-Induced Sleep Disorder[a]
                     Specify whether Insomnia type
F10.182   With mild use disorder
F10.282   With moderate or severe use disorder
F10.982   Without use disorder

___.__   Alcohol-Induced Sexual Dysfunction[a]
                     Specify if: Mild, Moderate, Severe
F10.181   With mild use disorder
F10.281   With moderate or severe use disorder
F10.981   Without use disorder

___.__   Alcohol Intoxication Delirium[b,c]
F10.121   With mild use disorder
F10.221   With moderate or severe use disorder
F10.921   Without use disorder

___.__   Alcohol Withdrawal Delirium[b,c]
F10.131   With mild use disorder
F10.231   With moderate or severe use disorder
F10.931   Without use disorder

___.__   Alcohol-Induced Major Neurocognitive Disorder
                     Specify if: Persistent
___.__   Amnestic-confabulatory type
F10.26   With moderate or severe use disorder
F10.96   Without use disorder
___.__   Nonamnestic-confabulatory type
F10.27   With moderate or severe use disorder
F10.97   Without use disorder

___.___   Alcohol-Induced Mild Neurocognitive Disorder
                  Specify if: Persistent
F10.188   With mild use disorder
F10.288   With moderate or severe use disorder
F10.988   Without use disorder

F10.99   Unspecified Alcohol-Related Disorder

Caffeine-Related Disorders

F15.920   Caffeine Intoxication

F15.93   Caffeine Withdrawal

___.___   Caffeine-Induced Mental Disorders
                  Note: Disorders are listed in their order of appearance in the
                      manual.
                  Specify With onset during intoxication, With onset during
                      withdrawal, With onset after medication use. **Note:** When
                      taken over the counter, substances in this class can also in-
                      duce the relevant substance-induced mental disorder.
F15.980   Caffeine-Induced Anxiety Disorder
F15.982   Caffeine-Induced Sleep Disorder
                      Specify whether Insomnia type, Daytime sleepiness type,
                      Mixed type

F15.99   Unspecified Caffeine-Related Disorder

Cannabis-Related Disorders

___.___   Cannabis Use Disorder
                  Specify if: In a controlled environment
                  Specify current severity/remission:
F12.10   Mild
F12.11   In early remission
F12.11   In sustained remission
F12.20   Moderate
F12.21   In early remission
F12.21   In sustained remission
F12.20   Severe
F12.21   In early remission
F12.21   In sustained remission

___.__	Cannabis Intoxication
	Without perceptual disturbances
F12.120	With mild use disorder
F12.220	With moderate or severe use disorder
F12.920	Without use disorder
	With perceptual disturbances
F12.122	With mild use disorder
F12.222	With moderate or severe use disorder
F12.922	Without use disorder
___.__	Cannabis Withdrawal
F12.13	With mild use disorder
F12.23	With moderate or severe use disorder
F12.93	Without use disorder
___.__	Cannabis-Induced Mental Disorders

Note: Disorders are listed in their order of appearance in the manual.

[a]*Specify* With onset during intoxication, With onset during withdrawal, With onset after medication use. **Note:** When prescribed as medication, substances in this class can also induce the relevant substance-induced mental disorder.

[b]*Specify* if: Acute, Persistent

[c]*Specify* if: Hyperactive, Hypoactive, Mixed level of activity

___.__	Cannabis-Induced Psychotic Disorder[a]
F12.159	With mild use disorder
F12.259	With moderate or severe use disorder
F12.959	Without use disorder
___.__	Cannabis-Induced Anxiety Disorder[a]
F12.180	With mild use disorder
F12.280	With moderate or severe use disorder
F12.980	Without use disorder
___.__	Cannabis-Induced Sleep Disorder[a]

Specify whether Insomnia type, Daytime sleepiness type, Mixed type

F12.188	With mild use disorder
F12.288	With moderate or severe use disorder
F12.988	Without use disorder

___.___   Cannabis Intoxication Delirium[b,c]
F12.121   With mild use disorder
F12.221   With moderate or severe use disorder
F12.921   Without use disorder
F12.921   Pharmaceutical Cannabis Receptor Agonist–Induced Delirium[b,c]

> **Note:** When pharmaceutical cannabis receptor medication taken as prescribed. The designation "taken as prescribed" is used to differentiate medication-induced delirium from substance intoxication delirium.

F12.99   Unspecified Cannabis-Related Disorder

Hallucinogen-Related Disorders

___.___   Phencyclidine Use Disorder
     Specify if: In a controlled environment
     Specify current severity/remission:
F16.10   Mild
F16.11   In early remission
F16.11   In sustained remission
F16.20   Moderate
F16.21   In early remission
F16.21   In sustained remission
F16.20   Severe
F16.21   In early remission
F16.21   In sustained remission

___.___   Other Hallucinogen Use Disorder
     Specify the particular hallucinogen
     Specify if: In a controlled environment
     Specify current severity/remission:
F16.10   Mild
F16.11   In early remission
F16.11   In sustained remission
F16.20   Moderate
F16.21   In early remission
F16.21   In sustained remission
F16.20   Severe
F16.21   In early remission
F16.21   In sustained remission

___.__   Phencyclidine Intoxication
F16.120   With mild use disorder
F16.220   With moderate or severe use disorder
F16.920   Without use disorder

___.__   Other Hallucinogen Intoxication
F16.120   With mild use disorder
F16.220   With moderate or severe use disorder
F16.920   Without use disorder

F16.983   Hallucinogen Persisting Perception Disorder

___.__   Phencyclidine-Induced Mental Disorders
              Note: Disorders are listed in their order of appearance in the
                 manual.
              [a]*Specify* With onset during intoxication, With onset after med-
                 ication use. **Note:** When prescribed as medication, substances
                 in this class can also induce the relevant substance-induced
                 mental disorder.

___.__   Phencyclidine-Induced Psychotic Disorder[a]
F16.159   With mild use disorder
F16.259   With moderate or severe use disorder
F16.959   Without use disorder

___.__   Phencyclidine-Induced Bipolar and Related Disorder[a]
F16.14   With mild use disorder
F16.24   With moderate or severe use disorder
F16.94   Without use disorder

___.__   Phencyclidine-Induced Depressive Disorder[a]
F16.14   With mild use disorder
F16.24   With moderate or severe use disorder
F16.94   Without use disorder

___.__   Phencyclidine-Induced Anxiety Disorder[a]
F16.180   With mild use disorder
F16.280   With moderate or severe use disorder
F16.980   Without use disorder

___.__   Phencyclidine Intoxication Delirium
                    Specify if: Acute, Persistent
                    Specify if: Hyperactive, Hypoactive, Mixed level of activity
F16.121   With mild use disorder

F16.221	With moderate or severe use disorder
F16.921	Without use disorder
___.__	Hallucinogen-Induced Mental Disorders

Note: Disorders are listed in their order of appearance in the manual.

[a]*Specify* With onset during intoxication, With onset after medication use. **Note:** When prescribed as medication, substances in this class can also induce the relevant substance-induced mental disorder.

[b]*Specify* if: Acute, Persistent

[c]*Specify* if: Hyperactive, Hypoactive, Mixed level of activity

___.__	Other Hallucinogen–Induced Psychotic Disorder[a]
F16.159	With mild use disorder
F16.259	With moderate or severe use disorder
F16.959	Without use disorder
___.__	Other Hallucinogen–Induced Bipolar and Related Disorder[a]
F16.14	With mild use disorder
F16.24	With moderate or severe use disorder
F16.94	Without use disorder
___.__	Other Hallucinogen–Induced Depressive Disorder[a]
F16.14	With mild use disorder
F16.24	With moderate or severe use disorder
F16.94	Without use disorder
___.__	Other Hallucinogen-Induced Anxiety Disorder[a]
F16.180	With mild use disorder
F16.280	With moderate or severe use disorder
F16.980	Without use disorder
___.__	Other Hallucinogen Intoxication Delirium[b,c]
F16.121	With mild use disorder
F16.221	With moderate or severe use disorder
F16.921	Without use disorder
F16.921	Ketamine or Other Hallucinogen–Induced Delirium[b,c]

Note: When ketamine or other hallucinogen medication taken as prescribed. The designation "taken as prescribed" is used to differentiate medication-induced delirium from substance intoxication delirium.

F16.99   Unspecified Phencyclidine-Related Disorder

F16.99   Unspecified Hallucinogen-Related Disorder

Inhalant-Related Disorders

___.___   Inhalant Use Disorder
           Specify the particular inhalant
           Specify if: In a controlled environment
           Specify current severity/remission:
F18.10   Mild
F18.11   In early remission
F18.11   In sustained remission
F18.20   Moderate
F18.21   In early remission
F18.21   In sustained remission
F18.20   Severe
F18.21   In early remission
F18.21   In sustained remission

___.___   Inhalant Intoxication
F18.120   With mild use disorder
F18.220   With moderate or severe use disorder
F18.920   Without use disorder

___.___   Inhalant-Induced Mental Disorders
           Note: Disorders are listed in their order of appearance in the
               manual.
           [a]*Specify* With onset during intoxication
___.___   Inhalant-Induced Psychotic Disorder[a]
F18.159   With mild use disorder
F18.259   With moderate or severe use disorder
F18.959   Without use disorder
___.___   Inhalant-Induced Depressive Disorder[a]
F18.14   With mild use disorder
F18.24   With moderate or severe use disorder
F18.94   Without use disorder

___.__	Inhalant-Induced Anxiety Disorder[a]
F18.180	With mild use disorder
F18.280	With moderate or severe use disorder
F18.980	Without use disorder
___.__	Inhalant Intoxication Delirium

Specify if: Acute, Persistent
Specify if: Hyperactive, Hypoactive, Mixed level of activity

F18.121	With mild use disorder
F18.221	With moderate or severe use disorder
F18.921	Without use disorder
___.__	Inhalant-Induced Major Neurocognitive Disorder

Specify if: Persistent

F18.17	With mild use disorder
F18.27	With moderate or severe use disorder
F18.97	Without use disorder
___.__	Inhalant-Induced Mild Neurocognitive Disorder

Specify if: Persistent

F18.188	With mild use disorder
F18.288	With moderate or severe use disorder
F18.988	Without use disorder
F18.99	Unspecified Inhalant-Related Disorder

Opioid-Related Disorders

___.__	Opioid Use Disorder

Specify if: On maintenance therapy, In a controlled environment
Specify current severity/remission:

F11.10	Mild
F11.11	In early remission
F11.11	In sustained remission
F11.20	Moderate
F11.21	In early remission
F11.21	In sustained remission
F11.20	Severe
F11.21	In early remission
F11.21	In sustained remission

___.__   Opioid Intoxication
                    Without perceptual disturbances
F11.120   With mild use disorder
F11.220   With moderate or severe use disorder
F11.920   Without use disorder
                    With perceptual disturbances
F11.122   With mild use disorder
F11.222   With moderate or severe use disorder
F11.922   Without use disorder

___.__   Opioid Withdrawal
F11.13   With mild use disorder
F11.23   With moderate or severe use disorder
F11.93   Without use disorder

___.__   Opioid-Induced Mental Disorders
                Note: Disorders are listed in their order of appearance in the
                    manual.
                [a]*Specify* With onset during intoxication, With onset during
                    withdrawal, With onset after medication use. **Note:** When
                    prescribed as medication, substances in this class can also
                    induce the relevant substance-induced mental disorder.
                [b]*Specify* if: Acute, Persistent
                [c]*Specify* if: Hyperactive, Hypoactive, Mixed level of activity
___.__   Opioid-Induced Depressive Disorder[a]
F11.14   With mild use disorder
F11.24   With moderate or severe use disorder
F11.94   Without use disorder
___.__   Opioid-Induced Anxiety Disorder[a]
F11.188   With mild use disorder
F11.288   With moderate or severe use disorder
F11.988   Without use disorder
___.__   Opioid-Induced Sleep Disorder[a]
                    Specify whether Insomnia type, Daytime sleepiness type,
                        Mixed type
F11.182   With mild use disorder
F11.282   With moderate or severe use disorder
F11.982   Without use disorder

___.__	Opioid-Induced Sexual Dysfunction[a]
	Specify if: Mild, Moderate, Severe
F11.181	With mild use disorder
F11.281	With moderate or severe use disorder
F11.981	Without use disorder
___.__	Opioid Intoxication Delirium[b,c]
F11.121	With mild use disorder
F11.221	With moderate or severe use disorder
F11.921	Without use disorder
___.__	Opioid Withdrawal Delirium[b,c]
F11.188	With mild use disorder
F11.288	With moderate or severe use disorder
F11.988	Without use disorder
___.__	Opioid-Induced Delirium[b,c]

Note: The designation "taken as prescribed" is used to differentiate medication-induced delirium from substance intoxication delirium and substance withdrawal delirium.

F11.921	When opioid medication taken as prescribed
F11.988	During withdrawal from opioid medication taken as prescribed
F11.99	Unspecified Opioid-Related Disorder

Sedative-, Hypnotic-, or Anxiolytic-Related Disorders

___.__	Sedative, Hypnotic, or Anxiolytic Use Disorder
	Specify if: In a controlled environment
	Specify current severity/remission:
F13.10	Mild
F13.11	In early remission
F13.11	In sustained remission
F13.20	Moderate
F13.21	In early remission
F13.21	In sustained remission
F13.20	Severe
F13.21	In early remission
F13.21	In sustained remission

___.__	Sedative, Hypnotic, or Anxiolytic Intoxication
F13.120	With mild use disorder
F13.220	With moderate or severe use disorder
F13.920	Without use disorder
___.__	Sedative, Hypnotic, or Anxiolytic Withdrawal
	Without perceptual disturbances
F13.130	With mild use disorder
F13.230	With moderate or severe use disorder
F13.930	Without use disorder
	With perceptual disturbances
F13.132	With mild use disorder
F13.232	With moderate or severe use disorder
F13.932	Without use disorder

___.__   Sedative-, Hypnotic-, or Anxiolytic-Induced Mental
            Disorders

Note: Disorders are listed in their order of appearance in the
    manual.

[a]*Specify* With onset during intoxication, With onset during
    withdrawal, With onset after medication use. **Note:** When
    prescribed as medication, substances in this class can also
    induce the relevant substance-induced mental disorder.

[b]*Specify* if: Acute, Persistent

[c]*Specify* if: Hyperactive, Hypoactive, Mixed level of activity

___.__	Sedative-, Hypnotic-, or Anxiolytic-Induced Psychotic Disorder[a]
F13.159	With mild use disorder
F13.259	With moderate or severe use disorder
F13.959	Without use disorder
___.__	Sedative-, Hypnotic-, or Anxiolytic-Induced Bipolar and Related Disorder[a]
F13.14	With mild use disorder
F13.24	With moderate or severe use disorder
F13.94	Without use disorder
___.__	Sedative-, Hypnotic-, or Anxiolytic-Induced Depressive Disorder[a]
F13.14	With mild use disorder
F13.24	With moderate or severe use disorder
F13.94	Without use disorder

___.___   Sedative-, Hypnotic-, or Anxiolytic-Induced Anxiety
                    Disorder[a]
F13.180   With mild use disorder
F13.280   With moderate or severe use disorder
F13.980   Without use disorder

___.___   Sedative-, Hypnotic-, or Anxiolytic-Induced Sleep
                    Disorder[a]
                 Specify whether Insomnia type, Daytime sleepiness type,
                    Parasomnia type, Mixed type
F13.182   With mild use disorder
F13.282   With moderate or severe use disorder
F13.982   Without use disorder

___.___   Sedative-, Hypnotic-, or Anxiolytic-Induced Sexual
                    Dysfunction[a]
                 Specify if: Mild, Moderate, Severe
F13.181   With mild use disorder
F13.281   With moderate or severe use disorder
F13.981   Without use disorder

___.___   Sedative-, Hypnotic-, or Anxiolytic Intoxication
                    Delirium[b,c]
F13.121   With mild use disorder
F13.221   With moderate or severe use disorder
F13.921   Without use disorder

___.___   Sedative-, Hypnotic-, or Anxiolytic Withdrawal
                    Delirium[b,c]
F13.131   With mild use disorder
F13.231   With moderate or severe use disorder
F13.931   Without use disorder

___.___   Sedative-, Hypnotic-, or Anxiolytic-Induced
                    Delirium[b,c]
                 Note: The designation "taken as prescribed" is used to differ-
                    entiate medication-induced delirium from substance in-
                    toxication delirium and substance withdrawal delirium.
F13.921   When sedative, hypnotic, or anxiolytic medication
                    taken as prescribed
F13.931   During withdrawal from sedative, hypnotic, or
                    anxiolytic medication taken as prescribed

___.___   Sedative-, Hypnotic-, or Anxiolytic-Induced Major
                   Neurocognitive Disorder
               Specify if: Persistent
F13.27   With moderate or severe use disorder
F13.97   Without use disorder

___.___   Sedative-, Hypnotic-, or Anxiolytic-Induced Mild
                   Neurocognitive Disorder
               Specify if: Persistent
F13.188   With mild use disorder
F13.288   With moderate or severe use disorder
F13.988   Without use disorder

F13.99   Unspecified Sedative-, Hypnotic-, or Anxiolytic-Related
               Disorder

Stimulant-Related Disorders

___.___   Stimulant Use Disorder
               Specify if: In a controlled environment
               Specify current severity/remission:
___.___   Mild
F15.10   Amphetamine-type substance
F14.10   Cocaine
F15.10   Other or unspecified stimulant
___.___   Mild, In early remission
F15.11   Amphetamine-type substance
F14.11   Cocaine
F15.11   Other or unspecified stimulant
___.___   Mild, In sustained remission
F15.11   Amphetamine-type substance
F14.11   Cocaine
F15.11   Other or unspecified stimulant
___.___   Moderate
F15.20   Amphetamine-type substance
F14.20   Cocaine
F15.20   Other or unspecified stimulant
___.___   Moderate, In early remission
F15.21   Amphetamine-type substance
F14.21   Cocaine
F15.21   Other or unspecified stimulant

___.__	Moderate, In sustained remission
F15.21	Amphetamine-type substance
F14.21	Cocaine
F15.21	Other or unspecified stimulant
___.__	Severe
F15.20	Amphetamine-type substance
F14.20	Cocaine
F15.20	Other or unspecified stimulant
___.__	Severe, In early remission
F15.21	Amphetamine-type substance
F14.21	Cocaine
F15.21	Other or unspecified stimulant
___.__	Severe, In sustained remission
F15.21	Amphetamine-type substance
F14.21	Cocaine
F15.21	Other or unspecified stimulant

___.__ Stimulant Intoxication
Specify the particular intoxicant
Without perceptual disturbances

___.__	Amphetamine-type substance or other stimulant intoxication
F15.120	With mild use disorder
F15.220	With moderate or severe use disorder
F15.920	Without use disorder
___.__	Cocaine intoxication
F14.120	With mild use disorder
F14.220	With moderate or severe use disorder
F14.920	Without use disorder

With perceptual disturbances

___.__	Amphetamine-type substance or other stimulant intoxication
F15.122	With mild use disorder
F15.222	With moderate or severe use disorder
F15.922	Without use disorder
___.__	Cocaine intoxication
F14.122	With mild use disorder
F14.222	With moderate or severe use disorder
F14.922	Without use disorder

___.__   Stimulant Withdrawal
   Specify the particular substance that causes the withdrawal syndrome

___.__   Amphetamine-type substance or other stimulant withdrawal
F15.13   With mild use disorder
F15.23   With moderate or severe use disorder
F15.93   Without use disorder

___.__   Cocaine withdrawal
F14.13   With mild use disorder
F14.23   With moderate or severe use disorder
F14.93   Without use disorder

___.__   Stimulant-Induced Mental Disorders
   Note: Disorders are listed in their order of appearance in the manual.
   [a]*Specify* With onset during intoxication, With onset during withdrawal, With onset after medication use. **Note:** When prescribed as medication, amphetamine-type substances and other stimulants can also induce the relevant substance-induced mental disorder.
   [b]*Specify* if: Acute, Persistent
   [c]*Specify* if: Hyperactive, Hypoactive, Mixed level of activity

___.__   Amphetamine-Type Substance (or Other Stimulant)–Induced Psychotic Disorder[a]
F15.159   With mild use disorder
F15.259   With moderate or severe use disorder
F15.959   Without use disorder

___.__   Cocaine-Induced Psychotic Disorder[a]
F14.159   With mild use disorder
F14.259   With moderate or severe use disorder
F14.959   Without use disorder

___.__   Amphetamine-Type Substance (or Other Stimulant)–Induced Bipolar and Related Disorder[a]
F15.14   With mild use disorder
F15.24   With moderate or severe use disorder
F15.94   Without use disorder

	Cocaine-Induced Bipolar and Related Disorder[a]
___.___	
F14.14	With mild use disorder
F14.24	With moderate or severe use disorder
F14.94	Without use disorder
___.___	Amphetamine-Type Substance (or Other Stimulant)–Induced Depressive Disorder[a]
F15.14	With mild use disorder
F15.24	With moderate or severe use disorder
F15.94	Without use disorder
___.___	Cocaine-Induced Depressive Disorder[a]
F14.14	With mild use disorder
F14.24	With moderate or severe use disorder
F14.94	Without use disorder
___.___	Amphetamine-Type Substance (or Other Stimulant)–Induced Anxiety Disorder[a]
F15.180	With mild use disorder
F15.280	With moderate or severe use disorder
F15.980	Without use disorder
___.___	Cocaine-Induced Anxiety Disorder[a]
F14.180	With mild use disorder
F14.280	With moderate or severe use disorder
F14.980	Without use disorder
___.___	Amphetamine-Type Substance (or Other Stimulant)–Induced Obsessive-Compulsive and Related Disorder[a]
F15.188	With mild use disorder
F15.288	With moderate or severe use disorder
F15.988	Without use disorder
___.___	Cocaine-Induced Obsessive-Compulsive and Related Disorder[a]
F14.188	With mild use disorder
F14.288	With moderate or severe use disorder
F14.988	Without use disorder
___.___	Amphetamine-Type Substance (or Other Stimulant)–Induced Sleep Disorder[a]
	Specify whether Insomnia type, Daytime sleepiness type, Mixed type

F15.182	With mild use disorder
F15.282	With moderate or severe use disorder
F15.982	Without use disorder
___.__	Cocaine-Induced Sleep Disorder[a]
	Specify whether Insomnia type, Daytime sleepiness type, Mixed type
F14.182	With mild use disorder
F14.282	With moderate or severe use disorder
F14.982	Without use disorder
___.__	Amphetamine-Type Substance (or Other Stimulant)– Induced Sexual Dysfunction[a]
	Specify if: Mild, Moderate, Severe
F15.181	With mild use disorder
F15.281	With moderate or severe use disorder
F15.981	Without use disorder
___.__	Cocaine-Induced Sexual Dysfunction[a]
	Specify if: Mild, Moderate, Severe
F14.181	With mild use disorder
F14.281	With moderate or severe use disorder
F14.981	Without use disorder
___.__	Amphetamine-Type Substance (or Other Stimulant) Intoxication Delirium[b,c]
F15.121	With mild use disorder
F15.221	With moderate or severe use disorder
F15.921	Without use disorder
___.__	Cocaine Intoxication Delirium[b,c]
F14.121	With mild use disorder
F14.221	With moderate or severe use disorder
F14.921	Without use disorder
F15.921	Amphetamine-Type (or Other Stimulant) Medication– Induced Delirium[b,c]

Note: When amphetamine-type or other stimulant medication taken as prescribed. The designation "taken as prescribed" is used to differentiate medication-induced delirium from substance intoxication delirium.

___.___   Amphetamine-Type Substance (or Other Stimulant)–
Induced Mild Neurocognitive Disorder
Specify if: Persistent

F15.188   With mild use disorder

F15.288   With moderate or severe use disorder

F15.988   Without use disorder

___.___   Cocaine-Induced Mild Neurocognitive Disorder
Specify if: Persistent

F14.188   With mild use disorder

F14.288   With moderate or severe use disorder

F14.988   Without use disorder

___.___   Unspecified Stimulant-Related Disorder

F15.99   Amphetamine-type substance or other stimulant

F14.99   Cocaine

Tobacco-Related Disorders

___.___   Tobacco Use Disorder
Specify if: On maintenance therapy, In a controlled environment
Specify current severity/remission:

Z72.0   Mild

F17.200   Moderate

F17.201   In early remission

F17.201   In sustained remission

F17.200   Severe

F17.201   In early remission

F17.201   In sustained remission

F17.203   Tobacco Withdrawal
Note: The ICD-10-CM code indicates the comorbid presence of a moderate or severe tobacco use disorder, which must be present in order to apply the code for tobacco withdrawal.

___.__   Tobacco-Induced Mental Disorders

F17.208   Tobacco-Induced Sleep Disorder, With moderate or
                severe use disorder
                Specify whether Insomnia type, Daytime sleepiness type,
                Mixed type
                Specify With onset during withdrawal, With onset after
                medication use

F17.209   Unspecified Tobacco-Related Disorder

Other (or Unknown) Substance–Related Disorders

___.__   Other (or Unknown) Substance Use Disorder
                Specify if: In a controlled environment
                Specify current severity/remission:
F19.10   Mild
F19.11   In early remission
F19.11   In sustained remission
F19.20   Moderate
F19.21   In early remission
F19.21   In sustained remission
F19.20   Severe
F19.21   In early remission
F19.21   In sustained remission

___.__   Other (or Unknown) Substance Intoxication
                Without perceptual disturbances
F19.120   With mild use disorder
F19.220   With moderate or severe use disorder
F19.920   Without use disorder
                With perceptual disturbances
F19.122   With mild use disorder
F19.222   With moderate or severe use disorder
F19.922   Without use disorder

___.__   Other (or Unknown) Substance Withdrawal
                Without perceptual disturbances
F19.130   With mild use disorder
F19.230   With moderate or severe use disorder
F19.930   Without use disorder

With perceptual disturbances

F19.132   With mild use disorder
F19.232   With moderate or severe use disorder
F19.932   Without use disorder

___.___   Other (or Unknown) Substance–Induced Mental Disorders
Note: Disorders are listed in their order of appearance in the manual.

[a]*Specify* With onset during intoxication, With onset during withdrawal, With onset after medication use. **Note:** When prescribed as medication or taken over the counter, substances in this class can also induce the relevant substance-induced mental disorder.

[b]*Specify* if: Acute, Persistent

[c]*Specify* if: Hyperactive, Hypoactive, Mixed level of activity

___.___   Other (or Unknown) Substance–Induced Psychotic Disorder[a]
F19.159   With mild use disorder
F19.259   With moderate or severe use disorder
F19.959   Without use disorder

___.___   Other (or Unknown) Substance–Induced Bipolar and Related Disorder[a]
F19.14   With mild use disorder
F19.24   With moderate or severe use disorder
F19.94   Without use disorder

___.___   Other (or Unknown) Substance–Induced Depressive Disorder[a]
F19.14   With mild use disorder
F19.24   With moderate or severe use disorder
F19.94   Without use disorder

___.___   Other (or Unknown) Substance–Induced Anxiety Disorder[a]
F19.180   With mild use disorder
F19.280   With moderate or severe use disorder
F19.980   Without use disorder

___.___   Other (or Unknown) Substance–Induced Obsessive-Compulsive and Related Disorder[a]
F19.188   With mild use disorder
F19.288   With moderate or severe use disorder
F19.988   Without use disorder

___.__	Other (or Unknown) Substance–Induced Sleep Disorder[a]

Specify whether Insomnia type, Daytime sleepiness type, Parasomnia type, Mixed type

F19.182	With mild use disorder
F19.282	With moderate or severe use disorder
F19.982	Without use disorder
___.__	Other (or Unknown) Substance–Induced Sexual Dysfunction[a]

Specify if: Mild, Moderate, Severe

F19.181	With mild use disorder
F19.281	With moderate or severe use disorder
F19.981	Without use disorder
___.__	Other (or Unknown) Substance Intoxication Delirium[b,c]
F19.121	With mild use disorder
F19.221	With moderate or severe use disorder
F19.921	Without use disorder
___.__	Other (or Unknown) Substance Withdrawal Delirium[b,c]
F19.131	With mild use disorder
F19.231	With moderate or severe use disorder
F19.931	Without use disorder
___.__	Other (or Unknown) Medication–Induced Delirium[b,c]

Note: The designation "taken as prescribed" is used to differentiate medication-induced delirium from substance intoxication delirium and substance withdrawal delirium.

F19.921	When other (or unknown) medication taken as prescribed
F19.931	During withdrawal from other (or unknown) medication taken as prescribed
___.__	Other (or Unknown) Substance–Induced Major Neurocognitive Disorder

Specify if: Persistent

F19.17	With mild use disorder
F19.27	With moderate or severe use disorder
F19.97	Without use disorder

___.__   Other (or Unknown) Substance–Induced Mild
        Neurocognitive Disorder
       Specify if: Persistent

F19.188   With mild use disorder
F19.288   With moderate or severe use disorder
F19.988   Without use disorder

F19.99   Unspecified Other (or Unknown) Substance–Related
       Disorder

Non-Substance-Related Disorders

F63.0   Gambling Disorder
      Specify if: Episodic, Persistent
      Specify if: In early remission, In sustained remission
      Specify current severity: Mild, Moderate, Severe

Neurocognitive Disorders

___.__   Delirium
      Specify if: Acute, Persistent
      Specify if: Hyperactive, Hypoactive, Mixed level of activity
      [a]**Note:** For applicable ICD-10-CM codes, refer to the substance
        classes under Substance-Related and Addictive Disorders
        for the specific substance/medication-induced delirium.
        See also the criteria set and corresponding recording pro-
        cedures in the manual for more information.
      Specify whether:

___.__   Substance intoxication delirium[a]
___.__   Substance withdrawal delirium[a]
___.__   Medication-induced delirium[a]
F05   Delirium due to another medical condition
F05   Delirium due to multiple etiologies

F05   Other Specified Delirium
F05   Unspecified Delirium

Major and Mild Neurocognitive Disorders

Refer to the following sequence for coding and recording major and mild neurocognitive disorders (NCDs) in context with specific diagnoses listed, exceptions as noted:

Major and mild NCDs: *Specify* whether due to *[any of the following medical etiologies]*: Alzheimer's disease, Frontotemporal degeneration, Lewy body disease, Vascular disease, Traumatic brain injury, Substance/medication use, HIV infection, Prion disease, Parkinson's disease, Huntington's disease, Another medical condition, Multiple etiologies, Unknown etiology

Major and mild NCDs: Code first the *specific medical etiology* for the major or mild NCD. **Note:** No etiological medical code is used for major vascular NCD, major NCDs due to possible etiologies, substance/medication-induced major or mild NCD, or major or mild NCD due to unknown etiology.

[a]**Major NCD only:** Next code *severity* (placeholder "x" in 4th character of diagnostic codes below) as follows: .Ay mild, .By moderate, .Cy severe. **Note:** Not applicable to any substance/medication-induced NCD.

[b]**Major NCD only:** Then code any *accompanying behavioral or psychological disturbance* (placeholder "y" in 5th and 6th characters of diagnostic codes below): .x11 with agitation; .x4 with anxiety; .x3 with mood symptoms; .x2 with psychotic disturbance; .x18 with other behavioral or psychological disturbance (e.g., apathy); .x0 without accompanying behavioral or psychological disturbance. **Note:** In cases where there is more than one type of associated behavioral or psychological disturbance, each is coded separately.

[c]**Mild NCD only** *(exceptions: see note d below)*: Code either **F06.70** without behavioral disturbance or **F06.71** with behavioral disturbance (e.g., apathy, agitation, anxiety, mood symptoms, psychotic disturbance, or other behavioral symptoms). **Coding note for mild NCDs only:** Use additional disorder code(s) to indicate clinically significant psychiatric symptoms due to the same medical condition causing the mild NCD (e.g., F06.2 psychotic disorder due to Alzheimer's disease with delusions; F06.32 depressive disorder due to Parkinson's disease, with major depressive–like episode.) *Note:* The additional codes for mental disorders due to another medical condition are included with disorders with which they share phenomenology (e.g., for depressive disorders due to another medical condition, see "Depressive Disorders").

[d]**Mild NCD due to possible or unknown etiology:** Code only **G31.84**. No additional medical code is used. **Note:** "With behavioral disturbance" and "Without behavioral disturbance" cannot be coded but should still be recorded.

Major or Mild Neurocognitive Disorder Due to Alzheimer's Disease

F02.[xy]   Major Neurocognitive Disorder Due to Probable
              Alzheimer's Disease[a,b]
              Note: Code first **G30.9** Alzheimer's disease.

F03.[xy]   Major Neurocognitive Disorder Due to Possible
              Alzheimer's Disease[a,b]
              Note: No additional medical code.

___.___   Mild Neurocognitive Disorder Due to Probable
              Alzheimer's Disease[c]
              Note: Code first **G30.9** Alzheimer's disease.

F06.71   With behavioral disturbance

F06.70   Without behavioral disturbance

G31.84   Mild Neurocognitive Disorder Due to Possible
              Alzheimer's Disease[d]

Major or Mild Frontotemporal Neurocognitive Disorder

F02.[xy]   Major Neurocognitive Disorder Due to Probable
              Frontotemporal Degeneration[a,b]
              Note: Code first **G31.09** frontotemporal degeneration.

F03.[xy]   Major Neurocognitive Disorder Due to Possible
              Frontotemporal Degeneration[a,b]
              Note: No additional medical code.

___.___   Mild Neurocognitive Disorder Due to Probable
              Frontotemporal Degeneration[c]
              Note: Code first **G31.09** frontotemporal degeneration.

F06.71   With behavioral disturbance

F06.70   Without behavioral disturbance

G31.84   Mild Neurocognitive Disorder Due to Possible
              Frontotemporal Degeneration[d]

Major or Mild Neurocognitive Disorder With Lewy Bodies

F02.[xy] Major Neurocognitive Disorder With Probable Lewy
               Bodies[a,b]
               Note: Code first **G31.83** Lewy body disease.

F03.[xy] Major Neurocognitive Disorder With Possible Lewy
               Bodies[a,b]
               Note: No additional medical code.

___._   Mild Neurocognitive Disorder With Probable Lewy
               Bodies[c]
               Note: Code first **G31.83** Lewy body disease.

F06.71   With behavioral disturbance
F06.70   Without behavioral disturbance

G31.84   Mild Neurocognitive Disorder With Possible Lewy
               Bodies[d]

Major or Mild Vascular Neurocognitive Disorder

F01.[xy] Major Neurocognitive Disorder Probably Due to Vascular
               Disease[a,b]
               Note: No additional medical code.

F03.[xy] Major Neurocognitive Disorder Possibly Due to Vascular
               Disease[a,b]
               Note: No additional medical code.

___._   Mild Neurocognitive Disorder Probably Due to Vascular
               Disease[c]
               Note: Code first **I67.9** cerebrovascular disease.

F06.71   With behavioral disturbance
F06.70   Without behavioral disturbance

G31.84   Mild Neurocognitive Disorder Possibly Due to Vascular
               Disease[d]

Major or Mild Neurocognitive Disorder Due to Traumatic Brain Injury
Note: Code first **S06.2XAS** diffuse traumatic brain injury with loss of consciousness of unspecified duration, sequela.

F02.[xy] Major Neurocognitive Disorder Due to Traumatic Brain
               Injury[a,b]

___.___ Mild Neurocognitive Disorder Due to Traumatic Brain Injury[c]

F06.71   With behavioral disturbance

F06.70   Without behavioral disturbance

Substance/Medication-Induced Major or Mild Neurocognitive Disorder

Note: No additional medical code is used. For applicable ICD-10-CM codes, refer to the substance classes under Substance-Related and Addictive Disorders for the specific substance/medication-induced major or mild NCD. See also the criteria set and corresponding recording procedures in the manual for more information.

Coding note: The ICD-10-CM code depends on whether or not there is a comorbid substance use disorder present for the same class of substance. In any case, an additional separate diagnosis of a substance use disorder is not given. *Note:* The symptom specifiers "With agitation," "With anxiety," "With mood symptoms," "With psychotic disturbance," "With other behavioral or psychological disturbance," "Without accompanying behavioral or psychological disturbance" cannot be coded but should still be recorded.

Specify if: Persistent

___.___ Substance/Medication-Induced Major Neurocognitive Disorder
        Specify current NCD severity: Mild, Moderate, Severe

___.___ Substance/Medication-Induced Mild Neurocognitive Disorder

Major or Mild Neurocognitive Disorder Due to HIV Infection

Note: Code first **B20** HIV infection.

F02.[xy]   Major Neurocognitive Disorder Due to HIV Infection[a,b]

___.___ Mild Neurocognitive Disorder Due to HIV Infection[c]

F06.71   With behavioral disturbance

F06.70   Without behavioral disturbance

Major or Mild Neurocognitive Disorder Due to Prion Disease

Note: Code first **A81.9** prion disease.

F02.[xy]   Major Neurocognitive Disorder Due to Prion Disease[a,b]

___.__   Mild Neurocognitive Disorder Due to Prion Disease[c]
F06.71   With behavioral disturbance
F06.70   Without behavioral disturbance

Major or Mild Neurocognitive Disorder Due to Parkinson's Disease

F02.[xy]   Major Neurocognitive Disorder Probably Due to
             Parkinson's Disease[a,b]
             Note: Code first **G20.C** Parkinson's disease.

F03.[xy]   Major Neurocognitive Disorder Possibly Due to
             Parkinson's Disease[a,b]
             Note: No additional medical code.

___.__   Mild Neurocognitive Disorder Probably Due to
             Parkinson's Disease[c]
             Note: Code first **G20.C** Parkinson's disease.
F06.71   With behavioral disturbance
F06.70   Without behavioral disturbance

G31.84   Mild Neurocognitive Disorder Possibly Due to
             Parkinson's Disease[d]

Major or Mild Neurocognitive Disorder Due to Huntington's Disease
Note: Code first **G10** Huntington's disease.

F02.[xy]   Major Neurocognitive Disorder Due to Huntington's
             Disease[a,b]

___.__   Mild Neurocognitive Disorder Due to Huntington's
             Disease[c]
F06.71   With behavioral disturbance
F06.70   Without behavioral disturbance

Major or Mild Neurocognitive Disorder Due to Another Medical Condition
Note: Code first the other medical condition.

F02.[xy]   Major Neurocognitive Disorder Due to Another Medical
             Condition[a,b]

___.___   Mild Neurocognitive Disorder Due to Another Medical Condition[c]

F06.71   With behavioral disturbance

F06.70   Without behavioral disturbance

Major or Mild Neurocognitive Disorder Due to Multiple Etiologies

F02.[xy]   Major Neurocognitive Disorder Due to Multiple Etiologies[a,b]

         Note: Code first all the etiological medical conditions (with the exception of cerebrovascular disease, which is not coded). Then code **F02.[xy]**[a,b] once for major NCD due to all etiologies that apply. Code also **F01.[xy]**[a,b] for major NCD probably due to vascular disease, if present. Code also the relevant substance/medication-induced major NCDs if substances or medications play a role in the etiology.

___.___   Mild Neurocognitive Disorder Due to Multiple Etiologies[c]

         Note: Code first all the etiological medical conditions, including **I67.9** cerebrovascular disease, if present. Then code **F06.70** or **F06.71** once (see below for 5th character) for mild NCD due to all etiologies that apply, including mild NCD probably due to vascular disease, if present. Code also the relevant substance/medication-induced mild NCDs if substances or medications play a role in the etiology.

F06.71   With behavioral disturbance

F06.70   Without behavioral disturbance

Major or Mild Neurocognitive Disorder Due to Unknown Etiology

F03.[xy]   Major Neurocognitive Disorder Due to Unknown Etiology[a,b]

G31.84   Mild Neurocognitive Disorder Due to Unknown Etiology[d]

R41.9   Unspecified Neurocognitive Disorder

Note: No additional medical code.

Personality Disorders

Cluster A Personality Disorders

F60.0   Paranoid Personality Disorder

F60.1   Schizoid Personality Disorder

F21   Schizotypal Personality Disorder

Cluster B Personality Disorders

F60.2   Antisocial Personality Disorder

F60.3   Borderline Personality Disorder

F60.4   Histrionic Personality Disorder

F60.81   Narcissistic Personality Disorder

Cluster C Personality Disorders

F60.6   Avoidant Personality Disorder

F60.7   Dependent Personality Disorder

F60.5   Obsessive-Compulsive Personality Disorder

Other Personality Disorders

F07.0   Personality Change Due to Another Medical Condition
             Specify whether: Labile type, Disinhibited type, Aggressive
             type, Apathetic type, Paranoid type, Other type, Combined
             type, Unspecified type

F60.89   Other Specified Personality Disorder

F60.9   Unspecified Personality Disorder

Paraphilic Disorders

The following specifier applies to Paraphilic Disorders where indicated:
[a]*Specify* if: In a controlled environment, In full remission

F65.3   Voyeuristic Disorder[a]

F65.2   Exhibitionistic Disorder[a]

Specify whether: Sexually aroused by exposing genitals to pre-pubertal children, Sexually aroused by exposing genitals to physically mature individuals, Sexually aroused by exposing genitals to prepubertal children and to physically mature individuals

F65.81   Frotteuristic Disorder[a]

F65.51   Sexual Masochism Disorder[a]
Specify if: With asphyxiophilia

F65.52   Sexual Sadism Disorder[a]

F65.4   Pedophilic Disorder
Specify whether: Exclusive type, Nonexclusive type
Specify if: Sexually attracted to males, Sexually attracted to females, Sexually attracted to both
Specify if: Limited to incest

F65.0   Fetishistic Disorder[a]
Specify: Body part(s), Nonliving object(s), Other

F65.1   Transvestic Disorder[a]
Specify if: With fetishism, With autogynephilia

F65.89   Other Specified Paraphilic Disorder

F65.9   Unspecified Paraphilic Disorder

Other Mental Disorders and Additional Codes

F06.8   Other Specified Mental Disorder Due to Another Medical Condition

F09   Unspecified Mental Disorder Due to Another Medical Condition

F99   Other Specified Mental Disorder

F99   Unspecified Mental Disorder

Z03.89   No Diagnosis or Condition

Medication-Induced Movement Disorders and Other Adverse Effects of Medication

___.__	Medication-Induced Parkinsonism
G21.11	Antipsychotic Medication– and Other Dopamine Receptor Blocking Agent–Induced Parkinsonism
G21.19	Other Medication-Induced Parkinsonism
G21.0	Neuroleptic Malignant Syndrome
G24.02	Medication-Induced Acute Dystonia
G25.71	Medication-Induced Acute Akathisia
G24.01	Tardive Dyskinesia
G24.09	Tardive Dystonia
G25.71	Tardive Akathisia
G25.1	Medication-Induced Postural Tremor
G25.79	Other Medication-Induced Movement Disorder
___.__	Antidepressant Discontinuation Syndrome
T43.205A	Initial encounter
T43.205D	Subsequent encounter
T43.205S	Sequelae
___.__	Other Adverse Effect of Medication
T50.905A	Initial encounter
T50.905D	Subsequent encounter
T50.905S	Sequelae

Other Conditions That May Be a Focus of Clinical Attention

Suicidal Behavior and Nonsuicidal Self-Injury

Suicidal Behavior

___.__	Current Suicidal Behavior
T14.91XA	Initial encounter

T14.91XD   Subsequent encounter

Z91.51   History of Suicidal Behavior

Nonsuicidal Self-Injury

R45.88   Current Nonsuicidal Self-Injury

Z91.52   History of Nonsuicidal Self-Injury

Abuse and Neglect

Child Maltreatment and Neglect Problems

Child Physical Abuse

___.__   Child Physical Abuse, Confirmed

T74.12XA   Initial encounter

T74.12XD   Subsequent encounter

___.__   Child Physical Abuse, Suspected

T76.12XA   Initial encounter

T76.12XD   Subsequent encounter

___.__   Other Circumstances Related to Child Physical Abuse

Z69.010   Encounter for mental health services for victim of child physical abuse by parent

Z69.020   Encounter for mental health services for victim of nonparental child physical abuse

Z62.810   Personal history (past history) of physical abuse in childhood

Z69.011   Encounter for mental health services for perpetrator of parental child physical abuse

Z69.021   Encounter for mental health services for perpetrator of nonparental child physical abuse

Child Sexual Abuse

___.__   Child Sexual Abuse, Confirmed

T74.22XA   Initial encounter

T74.22XD   Subsequent encounter

___.__   Child Sexual Abuse, Suspected

T76.22XA   Initial encounter

T76.22XD   Subsequent encounter

___.__ Other Circumstances Related to Child Sexual Abuse

Z69.010 Encounter for mental health services for victim of child sexual abuse by parent

Z69.020 Encounter for mental health services for victim of nonparental child sexual abuse

Z62.810 Personal history (past history) of sexual abuse in childhood

Z69.011 Encounter for mental health services for perpetrator of parental child sexual abuse

Z69.021 Encounter for mental health services for perpetrator of nonparental child sexual abuse

Child Neglect

___.__ Child Neglect, Confirmed

T74.02XA Initial encounter

T74.02XD Subsequent encounter

___.__ Child Neglect, Suspected

T76.02XA Initial encounter

T76.02XD Subsequent encounter

___.__ Other Circumstances Related to Child Neglect

Z69.010 Encounter for mental health services for victim of child neglect by parent

Z69.020 Encounter for mental health services for victim of nonparental child neglect

Z62.812 Personal history (past history) of neglect in childhood

Z69.011 Encounter for mental health services for perpetrator of parental child neglect

Z69.021 Encounter for mental health services for perpetrator of nonparental child neglect

Child Psychological Abuse

___.__ Child Psychological Abuse, Confirmed

T74.32XA Initial encounter

T74.32XD Subsequent encounter

___.__ Child Psychological Abuse, Suspected

T76.32XA Initial encounter

T76.32XD Subsequent encounter

___.__ Other Circumstances Related to Child Psychological Abuse

Z69.010 Encounter for mental health services for victim of child psychological abuse by parent

Z69.020 Encounter for mental health services for victim of nonparental child psychological abuse

Z62.811 Personal history (past history) of psychological abuse in childhood

Z69.011 Encounter for mental health services for perpetrator of parental child psychological abuse

Z69.021 Encounter for mental health services for perpetrator of nonparental child psychological abuse

Adult Maltreatment and Neglect Problems

Spouse or Partner Violence, Physical

___.__ Spouse or Partner Violence, Physical, Confirmed

T74.11XA Initial encounter

T74.11XD Subsequent encounter

___.__ Spouse or Partner Violence, Physical, Suspected

T76.11XA Initial encounter

T76.11XD Subsequent encounter

___.__ Other Circumstances Related to Spouse or Partner Violence, Physical

Z69.11 Encounter for mental health services for victim of spouse or partner violence, physical

Z91.410 Personal history (past history) of spouse or partner violence, physical

Z69.12 Encounter for mental health services for perpetrator of spouse or partner violence, physical

Spouse or Partner Violence, Sexual

___.__ Spouse or Partner Violence, Sexual, Confirmed

T74.21XA Initial encounter

T74.21XD Subsequent encounter

___.__ Spouse or Partner Violence, Sexual, Suspected

T76.21XA Initial encounter

T76.21XD Subsequent encounter

___.__   Other Circumstances Related to Spouse or Partner
                  Violence, Sexual
Z69.81   Encounter for mental health services for victim of
                  spouse or partner violence, sexual
Z91.410   Personal history (past history) of spouse or partner
                  violence, sexual
Z69.12   Encounter for mental health services for perpetrator of
                  spouse or partner violence, sexual

Spouse or Partner Neglect

___.__   Spouse or Partner Neglect, Confirmed
T74.01XA Initial encounter
T74.01XD Subsequent encounter

___.__   Spouse or Partner Neglect, Suspected
T76.01XA Initial encounter
T76.01XD Subsequent encounter

___.__   Other Circumstances Related to Spouse or Partner Neglect
Z69.11   Encounter for mental health services for victim of
                  spouse or partner neglect
Z91.412   Personal history (past history) of spouse or partner
                  neglect
Z69.12   Encounter for mental health services for perpetrator of
                  spouse or partner neglect

Spouse or Partner Abuse, Psychological

___.__   Spouse or Partner Abuse, Psychological, Confirmed
T74.31XA Initial encounter
T74.31XD Subsequent encounter

___.__   Spouse or Partner Abuse, Psychological, Suspected
T76.31XA Initial encounter
T76.31XD Subsequent encounter

___.__   Other Circumstances Related to Spouse or Partner Abuse,
                  Psychological
Z69.11   Encounter for mental health services for victim of
                  spouse or partner psychological abuse
Z91.411   Personal history (past history) of spouse or partner
                  psychological abuse

Z69.12   Encounter for mental health services for perpetrator of spouse or partner psychological abuse

Adult Abuse by Nonspouse or Nonpartner

___.__   Adult Physical Abuse by Nonspouse or Nonpartner, Confirmed

T74.11XA   Initial encounter

T74.11XD   Subsequent encounter

___.__   Adult Physical Abuse by Nonspouse or Nonpartner, Suspected

T76.11XA   Initial encounter

T76.11XD   Subsequent encounter

___.__   Adult Sexual Abuse by Nonspouse or Nonpartner, Confirmed

T74.21XA   Initial encounter

T74.21XD   Subsequent encounter

___.__   Adult Sexual Abuse by Nonspouse or Nonpartner, Suspected

T76.21XA   Initial encounter

T76.21XD   Subsequent encounter

___.__   Adult Psychological Abuse by Nonspouse or Nonpartner, Confirmed

T74.31XA   Initial encounter

T74.31XD   Subsequent encounter

___.__   Adult Psychological Abuse by Nonspouse or Nonpartner, Suspected

T76.31XA   Initial encounter

T76.31XD   Subsequent encounter

___.__   Other Circumstances Related to Adult Abuse by Nonspouse or Nonpartner

Z69.81   Encounter for mental health services for victim of nonspousal or nonpartner adult abuse

Z69.82   Encounter for mental health services for perpetrator of nonspousal or nonpartner adult abuse

Relational Problems

___.___   Parent-Child Relational Problem
Z62.820   Parent–Biological Child
Z62.821   Parent–Adopted Child
Z62.822   Parent–Foster Child
Z62.898   Other Caregiver–Child

Z62.891   Sibling Relational Problem

Z63.0   Relationship Distress With Spouse or Intimate Partner

Problems Related to the Family Environment

Z62.29   Upbringing Away From Parents

Z62.898   Child Affected by Parental Relationship Distress

Z63.5   Disruption of Family by Separation or Divorce

Z63.8   High Expressed Emotion Level Within Family

Educational Problems

Z55.0   Illiteracy and Low-Level Literacy

Z55.1   Schooling Unavailable and Unattainable

Z55.2   Failed School Examinations

Z55.3   Underachievement in School

Z55.4   Educational Maladjustment and Discord With Teachers
              and Classmates

Z55.8   Problems Related to Inadequate Teaching

Z55.9   Other Problems Related to Education and Literacy

Occupational Problems

Z56.82   Problem Related to Current Military Deployment Status

Z56.0   Unemployment

Z56.1   Change of Job

Z56.2   Threat of Job Loss

Z56.3   Stressful Work Schedule

Z56.4	Discord With Boss and Workmates
Z56.5	Uncongenial Work Environment
Z56.6	Other Physical and Mental Strain Related to Work
Z56.81	Sexual Harassment on the Job
Z56.9	Other Problem Related to Employment

Housing Problems

Z59.01	Sheltered Homelessness
Z59.02	Unsheltered Homelessness
Z59.10	Inadequate Housing
Z59.2	Discord With Neighbor, Lodger, or Landlord
Z59.3	Problem Related to Living in a Residential Institution
Z59.9	Other Housing Problem

Economic Problems

Z59.41	Food Insecurity
Z58.6	Lack of Safe Drinking Water
Z59.5	Extreme Poverty
Z59.6	Low Income
Z59.7	Insufficient Social or Health Insurance or Welfare Support
Z59.9	Other Economic Problem

Problems Related to the Social Environment

Z60.2	Problem Related to Living Alone
Z60.3	Acculturation Difficulty
Z60.4	Social Exclusion or Rejection
Z60.5	Target of (Perceived) Adverse Discrimination or Persecution
Z60.9	Other Problem Related to Social Environment

Problems Related to Interaction With the Legal System

Z65.0   Conviction in Criminal Proceedings Without
             Imprisonment
Z65.1   Imprisonment or Other Incarceration
Z65.2   Problems Related to Release From Prison
Z65.3   Problems Related to Other Legal Circumstances

Problems Related to Other Psychosocial, Personal, and Environmental Circumstances

Z72.9   Problem Related to Lifestyle
Z64.0   Problems Related to Unwanted Pregnancy
Z64.1   Problems Related to Multiparity
Z64.4   Discord With Social Service Provider, Including Probation
             Officer, Case Manager, or Social Services Worker
Z65.4   Victim of Crime
Z65.4   Victim of Terrorism or Torture
Z65.5   Exposure to Disaster, War, or Other Hostilities

Problems Related to Access to Medical and Other Health Care

Z75.3   Unavailability or Inaccessibility of Health Care Facilities
Z75.4   Unavailability or Inaccessibility of Other Helping
             Agencies

Circumstances of Personal History

Z91.49   Personal History of Psychological Trauma
Z91.82   Personal History of Military Deployment

Other Health Service Encounters for Counseling and Medical Advice

Z31.5   Genetic Counseling
Z70.9   Sex Counseling

Z71.3   Dietary Counseling

Z71.9   Other Counseling or Consultation

Additional Conditions or Problems That May Be a Focus of Clinical Attention

Z91.83   Wandering Associated With a Mental Disorder

Z63.4   Uncomplicated Bereavement

Z60.0   Phase of Life Problem

Z65.8   Religious or Spiritual Problem

Z72.811   Adult Antisocial Behavior

Z72.810   Child or Adolescent Antisocial Behavior

Z91.199   Nonadherence to Medical Treatment

E66.9   Overweight or Obesity

Z76.5   Malingering

R41.81   Age-Related Cognitive Decline

R41.83   Borderline Intellectual Functioning

R45.89   Impairing Emotional Outbursts

Alphabetical Listing of DSM-5-TR Diagnoses and ICD-10-CM Codes

For periodic DSM-5-TR coding and other updates, see www.dsm5.org.

ICD-10-CM	Disorder, condition, or problem
Z60.3	Acculturation difficulty
F43.0	Acute stress disorder
	Adjustment disorders
F43.22	With anxiety
F43.21	With depressed mood
F43.24	With disturbance of conduct
F43.23	With mixed anxiety and depressed mood
F43.25	With mixed disturbance of emotions and conduct
F43.20	Unspecified
Z72.811	Adult antisocial behavior
F98.5	Adult-onset fluency disorder
	Adult physical abuse by nonspouse or nonpartner, Confirmed
T74.11XA	Initial encounter
T74.11XD	Subsequent encounter
	Adult physical abuse by nonspouse or nonpartner, Suspected
T76.11XA	Initial encounter
T76.11XD	Subsequent encounter

ICD-10-CM	Disorder, condition, or problem
	Adult psychological abuse by nonspouse or nonpartner, Confirmed
T74.31XA	Initial encounter
T74.31XD	Subsequent encounter
	Adult psychological abuse by nonspouse or nonpartner, Suspected
T76.31XA	Initial encounter
T76.31XD	Subsequent encounter
	Adult sexual abuse by nonspouse or nonpartner, Confirmed
T74.21XA	Initial encounter
T74.21XD	Subsequent encounter
	Adult sexual abuse by nonspouse or nonpartner, Suspected
T76.21XA	Initial encounter
T76.21XD	Subsequent encounter
R41.81	Age-related cognitive decline
F40.00	Agoraphobia
	Alcohol-induced anxiety disorder
F10.180	With mild use disorder
F10.280	With moderate or severe use disorder
F10.980	Without use disorder
	Alcohol-induced bipolar and related disorder
F10.14	With mild use disorder
F10.24	With moderate or severe use disorder
F10.94	Without use disorder
	Alcohol-induced depressive disorder
F10.14	With mild use disorder

ICD-10-CM   Disorder, condition, or problem

ICD-10-CM	Disorder, condition, or problem
F10.24	With moderate or severe use disorder
F10.94	Without use disorder
	Alcohol-induced major neurocognitive disorder, Amnestic-confabulatory type
F10.26	With moderate or severe use disorder
F10.96	Without use disorder
	Alcohol-induced major neurocognitive disorder, Nonamnestic-confabulatory type
F10.27	With moderate or severe use disorder
F10.97	Without use disorder
	Alcohol-induced mild neurocognitive disorder
F10.188	With mild use disorder
F10.288	With moderate or severe use disorder
F10.988	Without use disorder
	Alcohol-induced psychotic disorder
F10.159	With mild use disorder
F10.259	With moderate or severe use disorder
F10.959	Without use disorder
	Alcohol-induced sexual dysfunction
F10.181	With mild use disorder
F10.281	With moderate or severe use disorder
F10.981	Without use disorder
	Alcohol-induced sleep disorder
F10.182	With mild use disorder
F10.282	With moderate or severe use disorder
F10.982	Without use disorder
	Alcohol intoxication
F10.120	With mild use disorder

ICD-10-CM	Disorder, condition, or problem
F10.220	With moderate or severe use disorder
F10.920	Without use disorder
	Alcohol intoxication delirium
F10.121	With mild use disorder
F10.221	With moderate or severe use disorder
F10.921	Without use disorder
	Alcohol use disorder
F10.10	Mild
F10.11	In early remission
F10.11	In sustained remission
F10.20	Moderate
F10.21	In early remission
F10.21	In sustained remission
F10.20	Severe
F10.21	In early remission
F10.21	In sustained remission
	Alcohol withdrawal, With perceptual disturbances
F10.132	With mild use disorder
F10.232	With moderate or severe use disorder
F10.932	Without use disorder
	Alcohol withdrawal, Without perceptual disturbances
F10.130	With mild use disorder
F10.230	With moderate or severe use disorder
F10.930	Without use disorder
	Alcohol withdrawal delirium
F10.131	With mild use disorder
F10.231	With moderate or severe use disorder

ICD-10-CM Disorder, condition, or problem

F10.931	Without use disorder
F15.921	Amphetamine-type (or other stimulant) medication–induced delirium (amphetamine-type or other stimulant medication taken as prescribed)
	Amphetamine-type substance (or other stimulant)–induced anxiety disorder
F15.180	With mild use disorder
F15.280	With moderate or severe use disorder
F15.980	Without use disorder
	Amphetamine-type substance (or other stimulant)–induced bipolar and related disorder
F15.14	With mild use disorder
F15.24	With moderate or severe use disorder
F15.94	Without use disorder
	Amphetamine-type substance (or other stimulant)–induced depressive disorder
F15.14	With mild use disorder
F15.24	With moderate or severe use disorder
F15.94	Without use disorder
	Amphetamine-type substance (or other stimulant)–induced mild neurocognitive disorder
F15.188	With mild use disorder
F15.288	With moderate or severe use disorder
F15.988	Without use disorder
	Amphetamine-type substance (or other stimulant)–induced obsessive-compulsive and related disorder
F15.188	With mild use disorder
F15.288	With moderate or severe use disorder
F15.988	Without use disorder

ICD-10-CM	Disorder, condition, or problem
	Amphetamine-type substance (or other stimulant)–induced psychotic disorder
F15.159	With mild use disorder
F15.259	With moderate or severe use disorder
F15.959	Without use disorder
	Amphetamine-type substance (or other stimulant)–induced sexual dysfunction
F15.181	With mild use disorder
F15.281	With moderate or severe use disorder
F15.981	Without use disorder
	Amphetamine-type substance (or other stimulant)–induced sleep disorder
F15.182	With mild use disorder
F15.282	With moderate or severe use disorder
F15.982	Without use disorder
	Amphetamine-type substance intoxication
	Amphetamine-type substance intoxication, With perceptual disturbances
F15.122	With mild use disorder
F15.222	With moderate or severe use disorder
F15.922	Without use disorder
	Amphetamine-type substance intoxication, Without perceptual disturbances
F15.120	With mild use disorder
F15.220	With moderate or severe use disorder
F15.920	Without use disorder
	Amphetamine-type substance (or other stimulant) intoxication delirium
F15.121	With mild use disorder

ICD-10-CM	Disorder, condition, or problem
F15.221	With moderate or severe use disorder
F15.921	Without use disorder
	Amphetamine-type substance use disorder
F15.10	Mild
F15.11	In early remission
F15.11	In sustained remission
F15.20	Moderate
F15.21	In early remission
F15.21	In sustained remission
F15.20	Severe
F15.21	In early remission
F15.21	In sustained remission
	Amphetamine-type substance withdrawal
F15.13	With mild use disorder
F15.23	With moderate or severe use disorder
F15.93	Without use disorder
	Anorexia nervosa
F50.02	Binge-eating/purging type
F50.01	Restricting type
	Antidepressant discontinuation syndrome
T43.205A	Initial encounter
T43.205S	Sequelae
T43.205D	Subsequent encounter
G21.11	Antipsychotic medication– and other dopamine receptor blocking agent–induced parkinsonism
F60.2	Antisocial personality disorder
F06.4	Anxiety disorder due to another medical condition

ICD-10-CM	Disorder, condition, or problem
	Attention-deficit/hyperactivity disorder
F90.2	Combined presentation
F90.1	Predominantly hyperactive/impulsive presentation
F90.0	Predominantly inattentive presentation
F84.0	Autism spectrum disorder
F60.6	Avoidant personality disorder
F50.82	Avoidant/restrictive food intake disorder
F50.81	Binge-eating disorder
	Bipolar I disorder, Current or most recent episode depressed
F31.76	In full remission
F31.75	In partial remission
F31.31	Mild
F31.32	Moderate
F31.4	Severe
F31.5	With psychotic features
F31.9	Unspecified
F31.0	Bipolar I disorder, Current or most recent episode hypomanic
F31.72	In full remission
F31.71	In partial remission
F31.9	Unspecified
	Bipolar I disorder, Current or most recent episode manic
F31.74	In full remission
F31.73	In partial remission
F31.11	Mild
F31.12	Moderate

ICD-10-CM   Disorder, condition, or problem

ICD-10-CM	Disorder, condition, or problem
F31.13	Severe
F31.2	With psychotic features
F31.9	Unspecified
F31.9	Bipolar I disorder, Current or most recent episode unspecified
F31.81	Bipolar II disorder
	Bipolar and related disorder due to another medical condition
F06.33	With manic features
F06.33	With manic- or hypomanic-like episode
F06.34	With mixed features
F45.22	Body dysmorphic disorder
R41.83	Borderline intellectual functioning
F60.3	Borderline personality disorder
F23	Brief psychotic disorder
F50.2	Bulimia nervosa
F15.980	Caffeine-induced anxiety disorder, Without use disorder
F15.982	Caffeine-induced sleep disorder, Without use disorder
F15.920	Caffeine intoxication
F15.93	Caffeine withdrawal
	Cannabis-induced anxiety disorder
F12.180	With mild use disorder
F12.280	With moderate or severe use disorder
F12.980	Without use disorder
	Cannabis-induced psychotic disorder
F12.159	With mild use disorder

ICD-10-CM	Disorder, condition, or problem
F12.259	With moderate or severe use disorder
F12.959	Without use disorder
	Cannabis-induced sleep disorder
F12.188	With mild use disorder
F12.288	With moderate or severe use disorder
F12.988	Without use disorder
	Cannabis intoxication, With perceptual disturbances
F12.122	With mild use disorder
F12.222	With moderate or severe use disorder
F12.922	Without use disorder
	Cannabis intoxication, Without perceptual disturbances
F12.120	With mild use disorder
F12.220	With moderate or severe use disorder
F12.920	Without use disorder
	Cannabis intoxication delirium
F12.121	With mild use disorder
F12.221	With moderate or severe use disorder
F12.921	Without use disorder
F12.921	Cannabis receptor agonist–induced delirium, pharmaceutical (medication taken as prescribed)
	Cannabis use disorder
F12.10	Mild
F12.11	In early remission
F12.11	In sustained remission
F12.20	Moderate
F12.21	In early remission
F12.21	In sustained remission

ICD-10-CM Disorder, condition, or problem

ICD-10-CM	Disorder, condition, or problem
F12.20	Severe
F12.21	In early remission
F12.21	In sustained remission
	Cannabis withdrawal
F12.13	With mild use disorder
F12.23	With moderate or severe use disorder
F12.93	Without use disorder
F06.1	Catatonia associated with another mental disorder (catatonia specifier)
F06.1	Catatonic disorder due to another medical condition
	Central sleep apnea
G47.37	Central sleep apnea comorbid with opioid use
R06.3	Cheyne-Stokes breathing
G47.31	Idiopathic central sleep apnea
Z56.1	Change of job
Z72.810	Child or adolescent antisocial behavior
Z62.898	Child affected by parental relationship distress
F80.81	Childhood-onset fluency disorder (stuttering)
	Child neglect, Confirmed
T74.02XA	Initial encounter
T74.02XD	Subsequent encounter
	Child neglect, Suspected
T76.02XA	Initial encounter
T76.02XD	Subsequent encounter
	Child physical abuse, Confirmed
T74.12XA	Initial encounter
T74.12XD	Subsequent encounter

ICD-10-CM	Disorder, condition, or problem
	Child physical abuse, Suspected
T76.12XA	Initial encounter
T76.12XD	Subsequent encounter
	Child psychological abuse, Confirmed
T74.32XA	Initial encounter
T74.32XD	Subsequent encounter
	Child psychological abuse, Suspected
T76.32XA	Initial encounter
T76.32XD	Subsequent encounter
	Child sexual abuse, Confirmed
T74.22XA	Initial encounter
T74.22XD	Subsequent encounter
	Child sexual abuse, Suspected
T76.22XA	Initial encounter
T76.22XD	Subsequent encounter
	Circadian rhythm sleep-wake disorders
G47.22	Advanced sleep phase type
G47.21	Delayed sleep phase type
G47.23	Irregular sleep-wake type
G47.24	Non-24-hour sleep-wake type
G47.26	Shift work type
G47.20	Unspecified type
	Cocaine-induced anxiety disorder
F14.180	With mild use disorder
F14.280	With moderate or severe use disorder
F14.980	Without use disorder

ICD-10-CM   Disorder, condition, or problem

	Cocaine-induced bipolar and related disorder
F14.14	With mild use disorder
F14.24	With moderate or severe use disorder
F14.94	Without use disorder
	Cocaine-induced depressive disorder
F14.14	With mild use disorder
F14.24	With moderate or severe use disorder
F14.94	Without use disorder
	Cocaine-induced mild neurocognitive disorder
F14.188	With mild use disorder
F14.288	With moderate or severe use disorder
F14.988	Without use disorder
	Cocaine-induced obsessive-compulsive and related disorder
F14.188	With mild use disorder
F14.288	With moderate or severe use disorder
F14.988	Without use disorder
	Cocaine-induced psychotic disorder
F14.159	With mild use disorder
F14.259	With moderate or severe use disorder
F14.959	Without use disorder
	Cocaine-induced sexual dysfunction
F14.181	With mild use disorder
F14.281	With moderate or severe use disorder
F14.981	Without use disorder
	Cocaine-induced sleep disorder
F14.182	With mild use disorder
F14.282	With moderate or severe use disorder

ICD-10-CM	Disorder, condition, or problem
F14.982	Without use disorder
	Cocaine intoxication, With perceptual disturbances
F14.122	With mild use disorder
F14.222	With moderate or severe use disorder
F14.922	Without use disorder
	Cocaine intoxication, Without perceptual disturbances
F14.120	With mild use disorder
F14.220	With moderate or severe use disorder
F14.920	Without use disorder
	Cocaine intoxication delirium
F14.121	With mild use disorder
F14.221	With moderate or severe use disorder
F14.921	Without use disorder
	Cocaine use disorder
F14.10	Mild
F14.11	In early remission
F14.11	In sustained remission
F14.20	Moderate
F14.21	In early remission
F14.21	In sustained remission
F14.20	Severe
F14.21	In early remission
F14.21	In sustained remission
	Cocaine withdrawal
F14.13	With mild use disorder
F14.23	With moderate or severe use disorder
F14.93	Without use disorder

ICD-10-CM	Disorder, condition, or problem
	Conduct disorder
F91.2	Adolescent-onset type
F91.1	Childhood-onset type
F91.9	Unspecified onset
	Conversion disorder (*see* Functional neurological symptom disorder)
Z65.0	Conviction in civil or criminal proceedings without imprisonment
R45.88	Current nonsuicidal self-injury
	Current suicidal behavior
T14.91XA	Initial encounter
T14.91XD	Subsequent encounter
F34.0	Cyclothymic disorder
F52.32	Delayed ejaculation
	Delirium
F05	Delirium due to another medical condition
F05	Delirium due to multiple etiologies
	Medication-induced delirium (*see specific substances for codes*)
	Substance intoxication delirium (*see specific substances for codes*)
	Substance withdrawal delirium (*see specific substances for codes*)
F22	Delusional disorder
F60.7	Dependent personality disorder
F48.1	Depersonalization/derealization disorder
	Depressive disorder due to another medical condition
F06.31	With depressive features
F06.32	With major depressive–like episode

ICD-10-CM	Disorder, condition, or problem
F06.34	With mixed features
F82	Developmental coordination disorder
Z71.3	Dietary counseling
Z56.4	Discord with boss and workmates
Z59.2	Discord with neighbor, lodger, or landlord
Z64.4	Discord with social service provider, including probation officer, case manager, or social services worker
F94.2	Disinhibited social engagement disorder
Z63.5	Disruption of family by separation or divorce
F34.81	Disruptive mood dysregulation disorder
F44.0	Dissociative amnesia
F44.1	Dissociative amnesia, with dissociative fugue
F44.81	Dissociative identity disorder
Z55.4	Educational maladjustment and discord with teachers and classmates
F98.1	Encopresis
F98.0	Enuresis
F52.21	Erectile disorder
F42.4	Excoriation (skin-picking) disorder
F65.2	Exhibitionistic disorder
Z65.5	Exposure to disaster, war, or other hostilities
Z59.5	Extreme poverty
F68.A	Factitious disorder imposed on another
F68.10	Factitious disorder imposed on self
Z55.2	Failed school examination
F52.31	Female orgasmic disorder
F52.22	Female sexual interest/arousal disorder

ICD-10-CM	Disorder, condition, or problem
F65.0	Fetishistic disorder
Z59.41	Food insecurity
F65.81	Frotteuristic disorder
	Functional neurological symptom disorder (conversion disorder)
F44.4	With abnormal movement
F44.6	With anesthesia or sensory loss
F44.5	With attacks or seizures
F44.7	With mixed symptoms
F44.6	With special sensory symptom
F44.4	With speech symptom
F44.4	With swallowing symptoms
F44.4	With weakness/paralysis
F63.0	Gambling disorder
F64.0	Gender dysphoria in adolescents and adults
F64.2	Gender dysphoria in children
F41.1	Generalized anxiety disorder
Z31.5	Genetic counseling
F52.6	Genito-pelvic pain/penetration disorder
F88	Global developmental delay
F16.983	Hallucinogen persisting perception disorder
	For additional hallucinogen-related substance disorders and hallucinogen-induced mental disorders, see entries for Other hallucinogen and Phencyclidine
Z63.8	High expressed emotion level within family
Z91.52	History of nonsuicidal self-injury
Z91.51	History of suicidal behavior
F60.4	Histrionic personality disorder
F42.3	Hoarding disorder

ICD-10-CM	Disorder, condition, or problem
Z59.01	Homelessness, sheltered
Z59.02	Homelessness, unsheltered
F51.11	Hypersomnolence disorder
Z55.0	Illiteracy and low-level literacy
F45.21	Illness anxiety disorder
R45.89	Impairing emotional outbursts
Z65.1	Imprisonment or other incarceration
Z59.10	Inadequate housing
	Inhalant-induced anxiety disorder
F18.180	With mild use disorder
F18.280	With moderate or severe use disorder
F18.980	Without use disorder
	Inhalant-induced depressive disorder
F18.14	With mild use disorder
F18.24	With moderate or severe use disorder
F18.94	Without use disorder
	Inhalant-induced major neurocognitive disorder
F18.17	With mild use disorder
F18.27	With moderate or severe use disorder
F18.97	Without use disorder
	Inhalant-induced mild neurocognitive disorder
F18.188	With mild use disorder
F18.288	With moderate or severe use disorder
F18.988	Without use disorder
	Inhalant-induced psychotic disorder
F18.159	With mild use disorder
F18.259	With moderate or severe use disorder
F18.959	Without use disorder

ICD-10-CM	Disorder, condition, or problem
	Inhalant intoxication
F18.120	With mild use disorder
F18.220	With moderate or severe use disorder
F18.920	Without use disorder
	Inhalant intoxication delirium
F18.121	With mild use disorder
F18.221	With moderate or severe use disorder
F18.921	Without use disorder
	Inhalant use disorder
F18.10	Mild
F18.11	In early remission
F18.11	In sustained remission
F18.20	Moderate
F18.21	In early remission
F18.21	In sustained remission
F18.20	Severe
F18.21	In early remission
F18.21	In sustained remission
F51.01	Insomnia disorder
Z59.7	Insufficient social or health insurance or welfare support
	Intellectual developmental disorder (intellectual disability)
F70	Mild
F71	Moderate
F72	Severe
F73	Profound
F63.81	Intermittent explosive disorder

ICD-10-CM	Disorder, condition, or problem
F16.921	Ketamine or other hallucinogen–induced delirium (ketamine or other hallucinogen medication taken as prescribed or for medical reasons)
F63.2	Kleptomania
Z58.6	Lack of safe drinking water
F80.2	Language disorder
Z59.6	Low income
	Major depressive disorder, Recurrent episode
F33.42	In full remission
F33.41	In partial remission
F33.0	Mild
F33.1	Moderate
F33.2	Severe
F33.3	With psychotic features
F33.9	Unspecified
	Major depressive disorder, Single episode
F32.5	In full remission
F32.4	In partial remission
F32.0	Mild
F32.1	Moderate
F32.2	Severe
F32.3	With psychotic features
F32.9	Unspecified
___.___	Major frontotemporal neurocognitive disorder (*see* Major neurocognitive disorder due to possible frontotemporal degeneration; Major neurocognitive disorder due to probable frontotemporal degeneration)

ICD-10-CM   Disorder, condition, or problem

ICD-10-CM	Disorder, condition, or problem
___.___	Major neurocognitive disorder due to Alzheimer's disease (*see* Major neurocognitive disorder due to possible Alzheimer's disease; Major neurocognitive disorder due to probable Alzheimer's disease)
___.___	Major neurocognitive disorder due to possible Alzheimer's disease (*no additional medical code*)
___.___	Major neurocognitive disorder due to possible Alzheimer's disease, Mild (*no additional medical code*)
F03.A11	With agitation
F03.A4	With anxiety
F03.A3	With mood symptoms
F03.A2	With psychotic disturbance
F03.A18	With other behavioral or psychological disturbance
F03.A0	Without accompanying behavioral or psychological disturbance
___.___	Major neurocognitive disorder due to possible Alzheimer's disease, Moderate (*no additional medical code*)
F03.B11	With agitation
F03.B4	With anxiety
F03.B3	With mood symptoms
F03.B2	With psychotic disturbance
F03.B18	With other behavioral or psychological disturbance
F03.B0	Without accompanying behavioral or psychological disturbance
___.___	Major neurocognitive disorder due to possible Alzheimer's disease, Severe (*no additional medical code*)

ICD-10-CM   Disorder, condition, or problem

ICD-10-CM	Disorder, condition, or problem
F03.C11	With agitation
F03.C4	With anxiety
F03.C3	With mood symptoms
F03.C2	With psychotic disturbance
F03.C18	With other behavioral or psychological disturbance
F03.C0	Without accompanying behavioral or psychological disturbance
___.___	Major neurocognitive disorder due to possible Alzheimer's disease, Unspecified severity (*no additional medical code*)
F03.911	With agitation
F03.94	With anxiety
F03.93	With mood symptoms
F03.92	With psychotic disturbance
F03.918	With other behavioral or psychological disturbance
F03.90	Without accompanying behavioral or psychological disturbance
___.___	Major neurocognitive disorder due to probable Alzheimer's disease (*code first* G30.9 Alzheimer's disease)
___.___	Major neurocognitive disorder due to probable Alzheimer's disease, Mild (*code first* G30.9 Alzheimer's disease)
F02.A11	With agitation
F02.A4	With anxiety
F02.A3	With mood symptoms
F02.A2	With psychotic disturbance

ICD-10-CM   Disorder, condition, or problem

F02.A18	With other behavioral or psychological disturbance
F02.A0	Without accompanying behavioral or psychological disturbance
___.___	Major neurocognitive disorder due to probable Alzheimer's disease, Moderate (*code first* G30.9 Alzheimer's disease)
F02.B11	With agitation
F02.B4	With anxiety
F02.B3	With mood symptoms
F02.B2	With psychotic disturbance
F02.B18	With other behavioral or psychological disturbance
F02.B0	Without accompanying behavioral or psychological disturbance
___.___	Major neurocognitive disorder due to probable Alzheimer's disease, Severe (*code first* G30.9 Alzheimer's disease)
F02.C11	With agitation
F02.C4	With anxiety
F02.C3	With mood symptoms
F02.C2	With psychotic disturbance
F02.C18	With other behavioral or psychological disturbance
F02.C0	Without accompanying behavioral or psychological disturbance
___.___	Major neurocognitive disorder due to probable Alzheimer's disease, Unspecified severity (*code first* G30.9 Alzheimer's disease)
F02.811	With agitation

ICD-10-CM	Disorder, condition, or problem
F02.84	With anxiety
F02.83	With mood symptoms
F02.82	With psychotic disturbance
F02.818	With other behavioral or psychological disturbance
F02.80	Without accompanying behavioral or psychological disturbance
___.___	Major neurocognitive disorder due to another medical condition *(code first the other medical condition that applies)*
___.___	Major neurocognitive disorder due to another medical condition, Mild *(code first the other medical condition that applies)*
F02.A11	With agitation
F02.A4	With anxiety
F02.A3	With mood symptoms
F02.A2	With psychotic disturbance
F02.A18	With other behavioral or psychological disturbance
F02.A0	Without accompanying behavioral or psychological disturbance
___.___	Major neurocognitive disorder due to another medical condition, Moderate *(code first the other medical condition that applies)*
F02.B11	With agitation
F02.B4	With anxiety
F02.B3	With mood symptoms
F02.B2	With psychotic disturbance
F02.B18	With other behavioral or psychological disturbance

ICD-10-CM   Disorder, condition, or problem

F02.B0	Without accompanying behavioral or psychological disturbance
___.___	Major neurocognitive disorder due to another medical condition, Severe (*code first the other medical condition that applies*)
F02.C11	With agitation
F02.C4	With anxiety
F02.C3	With mood symptoms
F02.C2	With psychotic disturbance
F02.C18	With other behavioral or psychological disturbance
F02.C0	Without accompanying behavioral or psychological disturbance
___.___	Major neurocognitive disorder due to another medical condition, Unspecified severity (*code first the other medical condition that applies*)
F02.811	With agitation
F02.84	With anxiety
F02.83	With mood symptoms
F02.82	With psychotic disturbance
F02.818	With other behavioral or psychological disturbance
F02.80	Without accompanying behavioral or psychological disturbance
___.___	Major neurocognitive disorder due to possible frontotemporal degeneration (*no additional medical code*)
___.___	Major neurocognitive disorder due to possible frontotemporal degeneration, Mild (*no additional medical code*)
F03.A11	With agitation

ICD-10-CM   Disorder, condition, or problem

F03.A4	With anxiety
F03.A3	With mood symptoms
F03.A2	With psychotic disturbance
F03.A18	With other behavioral or psychological disturbance
F03.A0	Without accompanying behavioral or psychological disturbance
___.___	Major neurocognitive disorder due to possible frontotemporal degeneration, Moderate *(no additional medical code)*
F03.B11	With agitation
F03.B4	With anxiety
F03.B3	With mood symptoms
F03.B2	With psychotic disturbance
F03.B18	With other behavioral or psychological disturbance
F03.B0	Without accompanying behavioral or psychological disturbance
___.___	Major neurocognitive disorder due to possible frontotemporal degeneration, Severe *(no additional medical code)*
F03.C11	With agitation
F03.C4	With anxiety
F03.C3	With mood symptoms
F03.C2	With psychotic disturbance
F03.C18	With other behavioral or psychological disturbance
F03.C0	Without accompanying behavioral or psychological disturbance

ICD-10-CM   Disorder, condition, or problem

___.___	Major neurocognitive disorder due to possible frontotemporal degeneration, Unspecified severity *(no additional medical code)*
F03.911	With agitation
F03.94	With anxiety
F03.93	With mood symptoms
F03.92	With psychotic disturbance
F03.918	With other behavioral or psychological disturbance
F03.90	Without accompanying behavioral or psychological disturbance
___.___	Major neurocognitive disorder due to probable frontotemporal degeneration *(code first* G31.09 frontotemporal degeneration)
___.___	Major neurocognitive disorder due to probable frontotemporal degeneration, Mild *(code first* G31.09 frontotemporal degeneration)
F02.A11	With agitation
F02.A4	With anxiety
F02.A3	With mood symptoms
F02.A2	With psychotic disturbance
F02.A18	With other behavioral or psychological disturbance
F02.A0	Without accompanying behavioral or psychological disturbance
___.___	Major neurocognitive disorder due to probable frontotemporal degeneration, Moderate *(code first* G31.09 frontotemporal degeneration)
F02.B11	With agitation
F02.B4	With anxiety

ICD-10-CM	Disorder, condition, or problem
F02.B3	With mood symptoms
F02.B2	With psychotic disturbance
F02.B18	With other behavioral or psychological disturbance
F02.B0	Without accompanying behavioral or psychological disturbance
___.___	Major neurocognitive disorder due to probable frontotemporal degeneration, Severe (*code first* G31.09 frontotemporal degeneration)
F02.C11	With agitation
F02.C4	With anxiety
F02.C3	With mood symptoms
F02.C2	With psychotic disturbance
F02.C18	With other behavioral or psychological disturbance
F02.C0	Without accompanying behavioral or psychological disturbance
___.___	Major neurocognitive disorder due to probable frontotemporal degeneration, Unspecified severity (*code first* G31.09 frontotemporal degeneration)
F02.811	With agitation
F02.84	With anxiety
F02.83	With mood symptoms
F02.82	With psychotic disturbance
F02.818	With other behavioral or psychological disturbance
F02.80	Without accompanying behavioral or psychological disturbance
___.___	Major neurocognitive disorder due to HIV infection (*code first* B20 HIV infection)

ICD-10-CM   Disorder, condition, or problem

___.___	Major neurocognitive disorder due to HIV infection, Mild (*code first* B20 HIV infection)
F02.A11	With agitation
F02.A4	With anxiety
F02.A3	With mood symptoms
F02.A2	With psychotic disturbance
F02.A18	With other behavioral or psychological disturbance
F02.A0	Without accompanying behavioral or psychological disturbance
___.___	Major neurocognitive disorder due to HIV infection, Moderate (*code first* B20 HIV infection)
F02.B11	With agitation
F02.B4	With anxiety
F02.B3	With mood symptoms
F02.B2	With psychotic disturbance
F02.B18	With other behavioral or psychological disturbance
F02.B0	Without accompanying behavioral or psychological disturbance
___.___	Major neurocognitive disorder due to HIV infection, Severe (*code first* B20 HIV infection)
F02.C11	With agitation
F02.C4	With anxiety
F02.C3	With mood symptoms
F02.C2	With psychotic disturbance
F02.C18	With other behavioral or psychological disturbance
F02.C0	Without accompanying behavioral or psychological disturbance

ICD-10-CM	Disorder, condition, or problem
___.___	Major neurocognitive disorder due to HIV infection, Unspecified severity (*code first* B20 HIV infection)
F02.811	With agitation
F02.84	With anxiety
F02.83	With mood symptoms
F02.82	With psychotic disturbance
F02.818	With other behavioral or psychological disturbance
F02.80	Without accompanying behavioral or psychological disturbance
___.___	Major neurocognitive disorder due to Huntington's disease (*code first* G10 Huntington's disease)
___.___	Major neurocognitive disorder due to Huntington's disease, Mild (*code first* G10 Huntington's disease)
F02.A11	With agitation
F02.A4	With anxiety
F02.A3	With mood symptoms
F02.A2	With psychotic disturbance
F02.A18	With other behavioral or psychological disturbance
F02.A0	Without accompanying behavioral or psychological disturbance
___.___	Major neurocognitive disorder due to Huntington's disease, Moderate (*code first* G10 Huntington's disease)
F02.B11	With agitation
F02.B4	With anxiety
F02.B3	With mood symptoms

ICD-10-CM   Disorder, condition, or problem

F02.B2	With psychotic disturbance
F02.B18	With other behavioral or psychological disturbance
F02.B0	Without accompanying behavioral or psychological disturbance
___.___	Major neurocognitive disorder due to Huntington's disease, Severe (*code first* G10 Huntington's disease)
F02.C11	With agitation
F02.C4	With anxiety
F02.C3	With mood symptoms
F02.C2	With psychotic disturbance
F02.C18	With other behavioral or psychological disturbance
F02.C0	Without accompanying behavioral or psychological disturbance
___.___	Major neurocognitive disorder due to Huntington's disease, Unspecified severity (*code first* G10 Huntington's disease)
F02.811	With agitation
F02.84	With anxiety
F02.83	With mood symptoms
F02.82	With psychotic disturbance
F02.818	With other behavioral or psychological disturbance
F02.80	Without accompanying behavioral or psychological disturbance
___.___	Major neurocognitive disorder with Lewy bodies (*see* Major neurocognitive disorder with possible Lewy bodies; Major neurocognitive disorder with probable Lewy bodies)

ICD-10-CM   Disorder, condition, or problem

___.___	Major neurocognitive disorder with possible Lewy bodies *(no additional medical code)*
___.___	Major neurocognitive disorder with possible Lewy bodies, Mild *(no additional medical code)*
F03.A11	With agitation
F03.A4	With anxiety
F03.A3	With mood symptoms
F03.A2	With psychotic disturbance
F03.A18	With other behavioral or psychological disturbance
F03.A0	Without accompanying behavioral or psychological disturbance
___.___	Major neurocognitive disorder with possible Lewy bodies, Moderate *(no additional medical code)*
F03.B11	With agitation
F03.B4	With anxiety
F03.B3	With mood symptoms
F03.B2	With psychotic disturbance
F03.B18	With other behavioral or psychological disturbance
F03.B0	Without accompanying behavioral or psychological disturbance
___.___	Major neurocognitive disorder with possible Lewy bodies, Severe *(no additional medical code)*
F03.C11	With agitation
F03.C4	With anxiety
F03.C3	With mood symptoms
F03.C2	With psychotic disturbance
F03.C18	With other behavioral or psychological disturbance

ICD-10-CM   Disorder, condition, or problem

ICD-10-CM	Disorder, condition, or problem
F03.C0	Without accompanying behavioral or psychological disturbance
___.___	Major neurocognitive disorder with possible Lewy bodies, Unspecified severity (*no additional medical code*)
F03.911	With agitation
F03.94	With anxiety
F03.93	With mood symptoms
F03.92	With psychotic disturbance
F03.918	With other behavioral or psychological disturbance
F03.90	Without accompanying behavioral or psychological disturbance
___.___	Major neurocognitive disorder with probable Lewy bodies (*code first* G31.83 Lewy body disease)
___.___	Major neurocognitive disorder with probable Lewy bodies, Mild *code first* G31.83 Lewy body disease)
F02.A11	With agitation
F02.A4	With anxiety
F02.A3	With mood symptoms
F02.A2	With psychotic disturbance
F02.A18	With other behavioral or psychological disturbance
F02.A0	Without accompanying behavioral or psychological disturbance
___.___	Major neurocognitive disorder with probable Lewy bodies, Moderate (*code first* G31.83 Lewy body disease)
F02.B11	With agitation

ICD-10-CM   Disorder, condition, or problem

F02.B4	With anxiety
F02.B3	With mood symptoms
F02.B2	With psychotic disturbance
F02.B18	With other behavioral or psychological disturbance
F02.B0	Without accompanying behavioral or psychological disturbance
___.___	Major neurocognitive disorder with probable Lewy bodies, Severe (*code first* G31.83 Lewy body disease)
F02.C11	With agitation
F02.C4	With anxiety
F02.C3	With mood symptoms
F02.C2	With psychotic disturbance
F02.C18	With other behavioral or psychological disturbance
F02.C0	Without accompanying behavioral or psychological disturbance
___.___	Major neurocognitive disorder with probable Lewy bodies, Unspecified severity (*code first* G31.83 Lewy body disease)
F02.811	With agitation
F02.84	With anxiety
F02.83	With mood symptoms
F02.82	With psychotic disturbance
F02.818	With other behavioral or psychological disturbance
F02.80	Without accompanying behavioral or psychological disturbance

ICD-10-CM Disorder, condition, or problem

ICD-10-CM	Disorder, condition, or problem
___.___	Major neurocognitive disorder due to multiple etiologies *(code first the other medical etiologies)*
___.___	Major neurocognitive disorder due to multiple etiologies, Mild *(code first the other medical etiologies)*
F02.A11	With agitation
F02.A4	With anxiety
F02.A3	With mood symptoms
F02.A2	With psychotic disturbance
F02.A18	With other behavioral or psychological disturbance
F02.A0	Without accompanying behavioral or psychological disturbance
___.___	Major neurocognitive disorder due to multiple etiologies, Moderate *(code first the other medical etiologies)*
F02.B11	With agitation
F02.B4	With anxiety
F02.B3	With mood symptoms
F02.B2	With psychotic disturbance
F02.B18	With other behavioral or psychological disturbance
F02.B0	Without accompanying behavioral or psychological disturbance
___.___	Major neurocognitive disorder due to multiple etiologies, Severe *(code first the other medical etiologies)*
F02.C11	With agitation
F02.C4	With anxiety
F02.C3	With mood symptoms
F02.C2	With psychotic disturbance

ICD-10-CM	Disorder, condition, or problem
F02.C18	With other behavioral or psychological disturbance
F02.C0	Without accompanying behavioral or psychological disturbance
___.___	Major neurocognitive disorder due to multiple etiologies, Unspecified severity *(code first the other medical etiologies)*
F02.811	With agitation
F02.84	With anxiety
F02.83	With mood symptoms
F02.82	With psychotic disturbance
F02.818	With other behavioral or psychological disturbance
F02.80	Without accompanying behavioral or psychological disturbance
___.___	Major neurocognitive disorder due to Parkinson's disease *(see* Major neurocognitive disorder possibly due to Parkinson's disease; Major neurocognitive disorder probably due to Parkinson's disease*)*
___.___	Major neurocognitive disorder possibly due to Parkinson's disease *(no additional medical code)*
___.___	Major neurocognitive disorder possibly due to Parkinson's disease, Mild *(no additional medical code)*
F03.A11	With agitation
F03.A4	With anxiety
F03.A3	With mood symptoms
F03.A2	With psychotic disturbance
F03.A18	With other behavioral or psychological disturbance

ICD-10-CM   Disorder, condition, or problem

F03.A0	Without accompanying behavioral or psychological disturbance
___.___	Major neurocognitive disorder possibly due to Parkinson's disease, Moderate *(no additional medical code)*
F03.B11	With agitation
F03.B4	With anxiety
F03.B3	With mood symptoms
F03.B2	With psychotic disturbance
F03.B18	With other behavioral or psychological disturbance
F03.B0	Without accompanying behavioral or psychological disturbance
___.___	Major neurocognitive disorder possibly due to Parkinson's disease, Severe *(no additional medical code)*
F03.C11	With agitation
F03.C4	With anxiety
F03.C3	With mood symptoms
F03.C2	With psychotic disturbance
F03.C18	With other behavioral or psychological disturbance
F03.C0	Without accompanying behavioral or psychological disturbance
___.___	Major neurocognitive disorder possibly due to Parkinson's disease, Unspecified severity *(no additional medical code)*
F03.911	With agitation
F03.94	With anxiety
F03.93	With mood symptoms
F03.92	With psychotic disturbance

ICD-10-CM	Disorder, condition, or problem
F03.918	With other behavioral or psychological disturbance
F03.90	Without accompanying behavioral or psychological disturbance
___.___	Major neurocognitive disorder probably due to Parkinson's disease (*code first* G20.C Parkinson's disease)
___.___	Major neurocognitive disorder probably due to Parkinson's disease, Mild (*code first* G20.C Parkinson's disease)
F02.A11	With agitation
F02.A4	With anxiety
F02.A3	With mood symptoms
F02.A2	With psychotic disturbance
F02.A18	With other behavioral or psychological disturbance
F02.A0	Without accompanying behavioral or psychological disturbance
___.___	Major neurocognitive disorder probably due to Parkinson's disease, Moderate (*code first* G20.C Parkinson's disease)
F02.B11	With agitation
F02.B4	With anxiety
F02.B3	With mood symptoms
F02.B2	With psychotic disturbance
F02.B18	With other behavioral or psychological disturbance
F02.B0	Without accompanying behavioral or psychological disturbance

---

ICD-10-CM   Disorder, condition, or problem

___.___	Major neurocognitive disorder probably due to Parkinson's disease, Severe (*code first* G20.C Parkinson's disease)
F02.C11	With agitation
F02.C4	With anxiety
F02.C3	With mood symptoms
F02.C2	With psychotic disturbance
F02.C18	With other behavioral or psychological disturbance
F02.C0	Without accompanying behavioral or psychological disturbance
___.___	Major neurocognitive disorder probably due to Parkinson's disease, Unspecified severity (*code first* G20.C Parkinson's disease)
F02.811	With agitation
F02.84	With anxiety
F02.83	With mood symptoms
F02.82	With psychotic disturbance
F02.818	With other behavioral or psychological disturbance
F02.80	Without accompanying behavioral or psychological disturbance
___.___	Major neurocognitive disorder due to prion disease (*code first* A81.9 prion disease)
___.___	Major neurocognitive disorder due to prion disease, Mild (*code first* A81.9 prion disease)
F02.A11	With agitation
F02.A4	With anxiety
F02.A3	With mood symptoms
F02.A2	With psychotic disturbance

ICD-10-CM   Disorder, condition, or problem

F02.A18	With other behavioral or psychological disturbance
F02.A0	Without accompanying behavioral or psychological disturbance
___.___	Major neurocognitive disorder due to prion disease, Moderate (*code first* A81.9 prion disease)
F02.B11	With agitation
F02.B4	With anxiety
F02.B3	With mood symptoms
F02.B2	With psychotic disturbance
F02.B18	With other behavioral or psychological disturbance
F02.B0	Without accompanying behavioral or psychological disturbance
___.___	Major neurocognitive disorder due to prion disease, Severe (*code first* A81.9 prion disease)
F02.C11	With agitation
F02.C4	With anxiety
F02.C3	With mood symptoms
F02.C2	With psychotic disturbance
F02.C18	With other behavioral or psychological disturbance
F02.C0	Without accompanying behavioral or psychological disturbance
___.___	Major neurocognitive disorder due to prion disease, Unspecified severity (*code first* A81.9 prion disease)
F02.811	With agitation
F02.84	With anxiety
F02.83	With mood symptoms

ICD-10-CM   Disorder, condition, or problem

F02.82	With psychotic disturbance
F02.818	With other behavioral or psychological disturbance
F02.80	Without accompanying behavioral or psychological disturbance
___.___	Major neurocognitive disorder due to traumatic brain injury (*code first* S06.2XAS diffuse traumatic brain injury with loss of consciousness of unspecified duration, sequela)
___.___	Major neurocognitive disorder due to traumatic brain injury, Mild (*code first* S06.2XAS diffuse traumatic brain injury with loss of consciousness of unspecified duration, sequela)
F02.A11	With agitation
F02.A4	With anxiety
F02.A3	With mood symptoms
F02.A2	With psychotic disturbance
F02.A18	With other behavioral or psychological disturbance
F02.A0	Without accompanying behavioral or psychological disturbance
___.___	Major neurocognitive disorder due to traumatic brain injury, Moderate (*code first* S06.2XAS diffuse traumatic brain injury with loss of consciousness of unspecified duration, sequela)
F02.B11	With agitation
F02.B4	With anxiety
F02.B3	With mood symptoms
F02.B2	With psychotic disturbance
F02.B18	With other behavioral or psychological disturbance

ICD-10-CM	Disorder, condition, or problem
F02.B0	Without accompanying behavioral or psychological disturbance
___.___	Major neurocognitive disorder due to traumatic brain injury, Severe (*code first* S06.2XAS diffuse traumatic brain injury with loss of consciousness of unspecified duration, sequela)
F02.C11	With agitation
F02.C4	With anxiety
F02.C3	With mood symptoms
F02.C2	With psychotic disturbance
F02.C18	With other behavioral or psychological disturbance
F02.C0	Without accompanying behavioral or psychological disturbance
___.___	Major neurocognitive disorder due to traumatic brain injury, Unspecified severity (*code first* S06.2XAS diffuse traumatic brain injury with loss of consciousness of unspecified duration, sequela)
F02.811	With agitation
F02.84	With anxiety
F02.83	With mood symptoms
F02.82	With psychotic disturbance
F02.818	With other behavioral or psychological disturbance
F02.80	Without accompanying behavioral or psychological disturbance
___.___	Major neurocognitive disorder due to unknown etiology (*no additional medical code*)

ICD-10-CM   Disorder, condition, or problem

___.___	Major neurocognitive disorder due to unknown etiology, Mild *(no additional medical code)*
F03.A11	With agitation
F03.A4	With anxiety
F03.A3	With mood symptoms
F03.A2	With psychotic disturbance
F03.A18	With other behavioral or psychological disturbance
F03.A0	Without accompanying behavioral or psychological disturbance
___.___	Major neurocognitive disorder due to unknown etiology, Moderate *(no additional medical code)*
F03.B11	With agitation
F03.B4	With anxiety
F03.B3	With mood symptoms
F03.B2	With psychotic disturbance
F03.B18	With other behavioral or psychological disturbance
F03.B0	Without accompanying behavioral or psychological disturbance
___.___	Major neurocognitive disorder due to unknown etiology, Severe *(no additional medical code)*
F03.C11	With agitation
F03.C4	With anxiety
F03.C3	With mood symptoms
F03.C2	With psychotic disturbance
F03.C18	With other behavioral or psychological disturbance

ICD-10-CM   Disorder, condition, or problem

F03.C0	Without accompanying behavioral or psychological disturbance
___.___	Major neurocognitive disorder due to unknown etiology, Unspecified severity *(no additional medical code)*
F03.911	With agitation
F03.94	With anxiety
F03.93	With mood symptoms
F03.92	With psychotic disturbance
F03.918	With other behavioral or psychological disturbance
F03.90	Without accompanying behavioral or psychological disturbance
___.___	Major vascular neurocognitive disorder *(see* Major neurocognitive disorder possibly due to vascular disease; Major neurocognitive disorder probably due to vascular disease)
___.___	Major neurocognitive disorder possibly due to vascular disease *(no additional medical code)*
___.___	Major neurocognitive disorder possibly due to vascular disease, Mild *(no additional medical code)*
F03.A11	With agitation
F03.A4	With anxiety
F03.A3	With mood symptoms
F03.A2	With psychotic disturbance
F03.A18	With other behavioral or psychological disturbance
F03.A0	Without accompanying behavioral or psychological disturbance

ICD-10-CM   Disorder, condition, or problem

___.___	Major neurocognitive disorder possibly due to vascular disease, Moderate *(no additional medical code)*
F03.B11	With agitation
F03.B4	With anxiety
F03.B3	With mood symptoms
F03.B2	With psychotic disturbance
F03.B18	With other behavioral or psychological disturbance
F03.B0	Without accompanying behavioral or psychological disturbance
___.___	Major neurocognitive disorder possibly due to vascular disease, Severe *(no additional medical code)*
F03.C11	With agitation
F03.C4	With anxiety
F03.C3	With mood symptoms
F03.C2	With psychotic disturbance
F03.C18	With other behavioral or psychological disturbance
F03.C0	Without accompanying behavioral or psychological disturbance
___.___	Major neurocognitive disorder possibly due to vascular disease, Unspecified severity *(no additional medical code)*
F03.911	With agitation
F03.94	With anxiety
F03.93	With mood symptoms
F03.92	With psychotic disturbance

ICD-10-CM	Disorder, condition, or problem
F03.918	With other behavioral or psychological disturbance
F03.90	Without accompanying behavioral or psychological disturbance
___.___	Major neurocognitive disorder probably due to vascular disease *(no additional medical code)*
___.___	Major neurocognitive disorder probably due to vascular disease, Mild *(no additional medical code)*
F01.A11	With agitation
F01.A4	With anxiety
F01.A3	With mood symptoms
F01.A2	With psychotic disturbance
F01.A18	With other behavioral or psychological disturbance
F01.A0	Without accompanying behavioral or psychological disturbance
___.___	Major neurocognitive disorder probably due to vascular disease, Moderate *(no additional medical code)*
F01.B11	With agitation
F01.B4	With anxiety
F01.B3	With mood symptoms
F01.B2	With psychotic disturbance
F01.B18	With other behavioral or psychological disturbance
F01.B0	Without accompanying behavioral or psychological disturbance
___.___	Major neurocognitive disorder probably due to vascular disease, Severe *(no additional medical code)*

ICD-10-CM	Disorder, condition, or problem
F01.C11	With agitation
F01.C4	With anxiety
F01.C3	With mood symptoms
F01.C2	With psychotic disturbance
F01.C18	With other behavioral or psychological disturbance
F01.C0	Without accompanying behavioral or psychological disturbance
___.___	Major neurocognitive disorder probably due to vascular disease, Unspecified severity *(no additional medical code)*
F01.511	With agitation
F01.54	With anxiety
F01.53	With mood symptoms
F01.52	With psychotic disturbance
F01.518	With other behavioral or psychological disturbance
F01.50	Without accompanying behavioral or psychological disturbance
F52.0	Male hypoactive sexual desire disorder
Z76.5	Malingering
G25.71	Medication-induced acute akathisia
G24.02	Medication-induced acute dystonia
	Medication-induced delirium *(see specific substances for codes)*
G25.1	Medication-induced postural tremor

ICD-10-CM   Disorder, condition, or problem

___.___	Mild frontotemporal neurocognitive disorder (*see* Mild neurocognitive disorder due to possible frontotemporal degeneration; Mild neurocognitive disorder due to probable frontotemporal degeneration)
___.___	Mild neurocognitive disorder due to Alzheimer's disease (*see* Mild neurocognitive disorder due to possible Alzheimer's disease; Mild neurocognitive disorder due to probable Alzheimer's disease)
G31.84	Mild neurocognitive disorder due to possible Alzheimer's disease (*no additional medical code*)
F06.71	Mild neurocognitive disorder due to probable Alzheimer's disease (*code first* G30.9 Alzheimer's disease), With behavioral disturbance
F06.70	Mild neurocognitive disorder due to probable Alzheimer's disease (*code first* G30.9 Alzheimer's disease), Without behavioral disturbance
F06.71	Mild neurocognitive disorder due to another medical condition (*code first* the other medical condition), With behavioral disturbance
F06.70	Mild neurocognitive disorder due to another medical condition (*code first* the other medical condition), Without behavioral disturbance
___.___	Mild frontotemporal neurocognitive disorder (*see* Mild neurocognitive disorder due to possible frontotemporal degeneration; Mild neurocognitive disorder due to probable frontotemporal degeneration)
G31.84	Mild neurocognitive disorder due to possible frontotemporal degeneration (*no additional medical code*)

ICD-10-CM Disorder, condition, or problem

F06.71   Mild neurocognitive disorder due to probable frontotemporal degeneration (*code first* G31.09 frontotemporal degeneration), With behavioral disturbance

F06.70   Mild neurocognitive disorder due to probable frontotemporal degeneration (*code first* G31.09 frontotemporal degeneration), Without behavioral disturbance

F06.71   Mild neurocognitive disorder due to HIV infection (*code first* B20 HIV infection), With behavioral disturbance

F06.70   Mild neurocognitive disorder due to HIV infection (*code first* B20 HIV infection), Without behavioral disturbance

F06.71   Mild neurocognitive disorder due to Huntington's disease (*code first* G10 Huntington's disease), With behavioral disturbance

F06.70   Mild neurocognitive disorder due to Huntington's disease (*code first* G10 Huntington's disease), Without behavioral disturbance

___.___ Mild neurocognitive disorder with Lewy bodies (*see* Mild neurocognitive disorder with possible Lewy bodies; Mild neurocognitive disorder with probable Lewy bodies)

G31.84   Mild neurocognitive disorder with possible Lewy bodies (*no additional medical code*)

F06.71   Mild neurocognitive disorder with probable Lewy bodies (*code first* G31.83 Lewy body disease), With behavioral disturbance

F06.70   Mild neurocognitive disorder with probable Lewy bodies (*code first* G31.83 Lewy body disease), Without behavioral disturbance

ICD-10-CM	Disorder, condition, or problem
F06.71	Mild neurocognitive disorder due to multiple etiologies (*code first* the other medical etiologies), With behavioral disturbance
F06.70	Mild neurocognitive disorder due to multiple etiologies (*code first* the other medical etiologies), Without behavioral disturbance
___.___	Mild neurocognitive disorder due to Parkinson's disease (*see* Mild neurocognitive disorder possibly due to Parkinson's disease; Mild neurocognitive disorder probably due to Parkinson's disease)
G31.84	Mild neurocognitive disorder possibly due to Parkinson's disease (*no additional medical code*)
F06.71	Mild neurocognitive disorder probably due to Parkinson's disease (*code first* G20.C Parkinson's disease), With behavioral disturbance
F06.70	Mild neurocognitive disorder probably due to Parkinson's disease (*code first* G20.C Parkinson's disease), Without behavioral disturbance
F06.71	Mild neurocognitive disorder due to prion disease (*code first* A81.9 prion disease), With behavioral disturbance
F06.70	Mild neurocognitive disorder due to prion disease (*code first* A81.9 prion disease), Without behavioral disturbance
F06.71	Mild neurocognitive disorder due to traumatic brain injury (*code first* S06.2XAS diffuse traumatic brain injury with loss of consciousness of unspecified duration, sequela), With behavioral disturbance

ICD-10-CM   Disorder, condition, or problem

F06.70	Mild neurocognitive disorder due to traumatic brain injury (*code first* S06.2XAS diffuse traumatic brain injury with loss of consciousness of unspecified duration, sequela), Without behavioral disturbance
G31.84	Mild neurocognitive disorder due to unknown etiology (*no additional medical code*)
___.___	Mild vascular neurocognitive disorder (*see* Mild neurocognitive disorder possibly due to vascular disease; Mild neurocognitive disorder probably due to vascular disease)
G31.84	Mild neurocognitive disorder possibly due to vascular disease (*no additional medical code*)
F06.71	Mild neurocognitive disorder probably due to vascular disease (*code first* I67.9 for cerebrovascular disease), With behavioral disturbance
F06.70	Mild neurocognitive disorder probably due to vascular disease (*code first* I67.9 for cerebrovascular disease), Without behavioral disturbance
F60.81	Narcissistic personality disorder
	Narcolepsy
G47.411	Narcolepsy with cataplexy or hypocretin deficiency (type 1)
G47.421	Narcolepsy with cataplexy or hypocretin deficiency due to a medical condition
G47.419	Narcolepsy without cataplexy and either without hypocretin deficiency or hypocretin unmeasured (type 2)
G47.429	Narcolepsy without cataplexy and without hypocretin deficiency due to a medical condition
G21.0	Neuroleptic malignant syndrome
F51.5	Nightmare disorder

ICD-10-CM	Disorder, condition, or problem
Z03.89	No diagnosis or condition
Z91.199	Nonadherence to medical treatment
	Non–rapid eye movement sleep arousal disorders
F51.4	Sleep terror type
F51.3	Sleepwalking type
R45.88	Nonsuicidal self-injury, current
Z91.52	Nonsuicidal self-injury, history of
F42.2	Obsessive-compulsive disorder
F60.5	Obsessive-compulsive personality disorder
F06.8	Obsessive-compulsive and related disorder due to another medical condition
G47.33	Obstructive sleep apnea hypopnea
	Opioid-induced anxiety disorder
F11.188	With mild use disorder
F11.288	With moderate or severe use disorder
F11.988	Without use disorder
F11.921	Opioid-induced delirium (opioid medication taken as prescribed)
F11.988	Opioid-induced delirium (during withdrawal from opioid medication taken as prescribed)
	Opioid-induced depressive disorder
F11.14	With mild use disorder
F11.24	With moderate or severe use disorder
F11.94	Without use disorder
	Opioid-induced sexual dysfunction
F11.181	With mild use disorder
F11.281	With moderate or severe use disorder
F11.981	Without use disorder

ICD-10-CM	Disorder, condition, or problem
	Opioid-induced sleep disorder
F11.182	With mild use disorder
F11.282	With moderate or severe use disorder
F11.982	Without use disorder
	Opioid intoxication, With perceptual disturbances
F11.122	With mild use disorder
F11.222	With moderate or severe use disorder
F11.922	Without use disorder
	Opioid intoxication, Without perceptual disturbances
F11.120	With mild use disorder
F11.220	With moderate or severe use disorder
F11.920	Without use disorder
	Opioid intoxication delirium
F11.121	With mild use disorder
F11.221	With moderate or severe use disorder
F11.921	Without use disorder
	Opioid use disorder
F11.10	Mild
F11.11	In early remission
F11.11	In sustained remission
F11.20	Moderate
F11.21	In early remission
F11.21	In sustained remission
F11.20	Severe
F11.21	In early remission
F11.21	In sustained remission

ICD-10-CM	Disorder, condition, or problem
	Opioid withdrawal
F11.13	With mild use disorder
F11.23	With moderate or severe use disorder
F11.93	Without use disorder
	Opioid withdrawal delirium
F11.188	With mild use disorder
F11.288	With moderate or severe use disorder
F11.988	Without use disorder
F91.3	Oppositional defiant disorder
	Other adverse effect of medication
T50.905A	Initial encounter
T50.905S	Sequelae
T50.905D	Subsequent encounter
	Other circumstances related to adult abuse by nonspouse or nonpartner
Z69.82	Encounter for mental health services for perpetrator of nonspousal or nonpartner adult abuse
Z69.81	Encounter for mental health services for victim of nonspousal or nonpartner adult abuse
	Other circumstances related to child neglect
Z69.021	Encounter for mental health services for perpetrator of nonparental child neglect
Z69.011	Encounter for mental health services for perpetrator of parental child neglect
Z69.010	Encounter for mental health services for victim of child neglect by parent
Z69.020	Encounter for mental health services for victim of nonparental child neglect

ICD-10-CM	Disorder, condition, or problem
Z62.812	Personal history (past history) of neglect in childhood
	Other circumstances related to child physical abuse
Z69.021	Encounter for mental health services for perpetrator of nonparental child physical abuse
Z69.011	Encounter for mental health services for perpetrator of parental child physical abuse
Z69.010	Encounter for mental health services for victim of child physical abuse by parent
Z69.020	Encounter for mental health services for victim of nonparental child physical abuse
Z62.810	Personal history (past history) of physical abuse in childhood
	Other circumstances related to child psychological abuse
Z69.021	Encounter for mental health services for perpetrator of nonparental child psychological abuse
Z69.011	Encounter for mental health services for perpetrator of parental child psychological abuse
Z69.010	Encounter for mental health services for victim of child psychological abuse by parent
Z69.020	Encounter for mental health services for victim of nonparental child psychological abuse
Z62.811	Personal history (past history) of psychological abuse in childhood
	Other circumstances related to child sexual abuse
Z69.021	Encounter for mental health services for perpetrator of nonparental child sexual abuse
Z69.011	Encounter for mental health services for perpetrator of parental child sexual abuse

---

ICD-10-CM	Disorder, condition, or problem
Z69.010	Encounter for mental health services for victim of child sexual abuse by parent
Z69.020	Encounter for mental health services for victim of nonparental child sexual abuse
Z62.810	Personal history (past history) of sexual abuse in childhood
	Other circumstances related to spouse or partner abuse, Psychological
Z69.12	Encounter for mental health services for perpetrator of spouse or partner psychological abuse
Z69.11	Encounter for mental health services for victim of spouse or partner psychological abuse
Z91.411	Personal history (past history) of spouse or partner psychological abuse
	Other circumstances related to spouse or partner neglect
Z69.12	Encounter for mental health services for perpetrator of spouse or partner neglect
Z69.11	Encounter for mental health services for victim of spouse or partner neglect
Z91.412	Personal history (past history) of spouse or partner neglect
	Other circumstances related to spouse or partner violence, Physical
Z69.12	Encounter for mental health services for perpetrator of spouse or partner violence, Physical
Z69.11	Encounter for mental health services for victim of spouse or partner violence, Physical
Z91.410	Personal history (past history) of spouse or partner violence, Physical
	Other circumstances related to spouse or partner violence, Sexual

ICD-10-CM	Disorder, condition, or problem
Z69.12	Encounter for mental health services for perpetrator of spouse or partner violence, Sexual
Z69.81	Encounter for mental health services for victim of spouse or partner violence, Sexual
Z91.410	Personal history (past history) of spouse or partner violence, Sexual
Z71.9	Other counseling or consultation
Z59.9	Other economic problem
	Other hallucinogen–induced anxiety disorder
F16.180	With mild use disorder
F16.280	With moderate or severe use disorder
F16.980	Without use disorder
	Other hallucinogen–induced bipolar and related disorder
F16.14	With mild use disorder
F16.24	With moderate or severe use disorder
F16.94	Without use disorder
F16.921	Other hallucinogen–induced delirium (other hallucinogen medication taken as prescribed or for medical reasons)
	Other hallucinogen–induced depressive disorder
F16.14	With mild use disorder
F16.24	With moderate or severe use disorder
F16.94	Without use disorder
	Other hallucinogen–induced psychotic disorder
F16.159	With mild use disorder
F16.259	With moderate or severe use disorder
F16.959	Without use disorder
	Other hallucinogen intoxication

ICD-10-CM	Disorder, condition, or problem
F16.120	With mild use disorder
F16.220	With moderate or severe use disorder
F16.920	Without use disorder
	Other hallucinogen intoxication delirium
F16.121	With mild use disorder
F16.221	With moderate or severe use disorder
F16.921	Without use disorder
	Other hallucinogen use disorder
F16.10	Mild
F16.11	In early remission
F16.11	In sustained remission
F16.20	Moderate
F16.21	In early remission
F16.21	In sustained remission
F16.20	Severe
F16.21	In early remission
F16.21	In sustained remission
Z59.9	Other housing problem
G25.79	Other medication-induced movement disorder
G21.19	Other medication-induced parkinsonism
Z91.49	Other personal history of psychological trauma
Z91.89	Other personal risk factors
Z56.6	Other physical and mental strain related to work
Z56.9	Other problem related to employment
Z60.9	Other problem related to social environment
Z55.9	Other problems related to education and literacy
F41.8	Other specified anxiety disorder

ICD-10-CM	Disorder, condition, or problem
F90.8	Other specified attention-deficit/hyperactivity disorder
F31.89	Other specified bipolar and related disorder
F05	Other specified delirium
F32.89	Other specified depressive disorder
F91.8	Other specified disruptive, impulse-control, and conduct disorder
F44.89	Other specified dissociative disorder
	Other specified elimination disorder
R15.9	With fecal symptoms
N39.498	With urinary symptoms
F50.89	Other specified feeding or eating disorder
F64.8	Other specified gender dysphoria
G47.19	Other specified hypersomnolence disorder
G47.09	Other specified insomnia disorder
F99	Other specified mental disorder
F06.8	Other specified mental disorder due to another medical condition
F88	Other specified neurodevelopmental disorder
F42.8	Other specified obsessive-compulsive and related disorder
F65.89	Other specified paraphilic disorder
F60.89	Other specified personality disorder
F28	Other specified schizophrenia spectrum and other psychotic disorder
F52.8	Other specified sexual dysfunction
G47.8	Other specified sleep-wake disorder
F45.8	Other specified somatic symptom and related disorder

ICD-10-CM	Disorder, condition, or problem
F95.8	Other specified tic disorder
F43.89	Other specified trauma- and stressor-related disorder
	Other stimulant intoxication, With perceptual disturbances
F15.122	With mild use disorder
F15.222	With moderate or severe use disorder
F15.922	Without use disorder
	Other stimulant intoxication, Without perceptual disturbances
F15.120	With mild use disorder
F15.220	With moderate or severe use disorder
F15.920	Without use disorder
	See also Other or unspecified stimulant use disorder
	Other stimulant withdrawal
F15.13	With mild use disorder
F15.23	With moderate or severe use disorder
F15.93	Without use disorder
F19.921	Other (or unknown) medication–induced delirium (other [or unknown] medication taken as prescribed)
F19.931	Other (or unknown) medication–induced delirium (during withdrawal from other [or unknown] medication taken as prescribed)
	Other (or unknown) substance–induced anxiety disorder
F19.180	With mild use disorder
F19.280	With moderate or severe use disorder
F19.980	Without use disorder

ICD-10-CM Disorder, condition, or problem

	Other (or unknown) substance–induced bipolar and related disorder
F19.14	With mild use disorder
F19.24	With moderate or severe use disorder
F19.94	Without use disorder
	Other (or unknown) substance–induced depressive disorder
F19.14	With mild use disorder
F19.24	With moderate or severe use disorder
F19.94	Without use disorder
	Other (or unknown) substance–induced major neurocognitive disorder
F19.17	With mild use disorder
F19.27	With moderate or severe use disorder
F19.97	Without use disorder
	Other (or unknown) substance–induced mild neurocognitive disorder
F19.188	With mild use disorder
F19.288	With moderate or severe use disorder
F19.988	Without use disorder
	Other (or unknown) substance–induced obsessive-compulsive and related disorder
F19.188	With mild use disorder
F19.288	With moderate or severe use disorder
F19.988	Without use disorder
	Other (or unknown) substance–induced psychotic disorder
F19.159	With mild use disorder
F19.259	With moderate or severe use disorder

ICD-10-CM	Disorder, condition, or problem
F19.959	Without use disorder
	Other (or unknown) substance–induced sexual dysfunction
F19.181	With mild use disorder
F19.281	With moderate or severe use disorder
F19.981	Without use disorder
	Other (or unknown) substance–induced sleep disorder
F19.182	With mild use disorder
F19.282	With moderate or severe use disorder
F19.982	Without use disorder
	Other (or unknown) substance intoxication, With perceptual disturbances
F19.122	With mild use disorder
F19.222	With moderate or severe use disorder
F19.922	Without use disorder
	Other (or unknown) substance intoxication, Without perceptual disturbances
F19.120	With mild use disorder
F19.220	With moderate or severe use disorder
F19.920	Without use disorder
	Other (or unknown) substance intoxication delirium
F19.121	With mild use disorder
F19.221	With moderate or severe use disorder
F19.921	Without use disorder
	Other (or unknown) substance use disorder
F19.10	Mild
F19.11	In early remission

ICD-10-CM   Disorder, condition, or problem

ICD-10-CM	Disorder, condition, or problem
F19.11	In sustained remission
F19.20	Moderate
F19.21	In early remission
F19.21	In sustained remission
F19.20	Severe
F19.21	In early remission
F19.21	In sustained remission
	Other (or unknown) substance withdrawal, With perceptual disturbances
F19.132	With mild use disorder
F19.232	With moderate or severe use disorder
F19.932	Without use disorder
	Other (or unknown) substance withdrawal, Without perceptual disturbances
F19.130	With mild use disorder
F19.230	With moderate or severe use disorder
F19.930	Without use disorder
	Other (or unknown) substance withdrawal delirium
F19.131	With mild use disorder
F19.231	With moderate or severe use disorder
F19.931	Without use disorder
	Other or unspecified stimulant use disorder
F15.10	Mild
F15.11	In early remission
F15.11	In sustained remission
F15.20	Moderate
F15.21	In early remission
F15.21	In sustained remission

ICD-10-CM	Disorder, condition, or problem
F15.20	Severe
F15.21	In early remission
F15.21	In sustained remission
E66.9	Overweight or obesity
no code	Panic attack specifier
F41.0	Panic disorder
F60.0	Paranoid personality disorder
	Parent-child relational problem
Z62.821	Parent–adopted child
Z62.820	Parent–biological child
Z62.822	Parent–foster child
Z62.898	Other caregiver–child
F65.4	Pedophilic disorder
F95.1	Persistent (chronic) motor or vocal tic disorder
F34.1	Persistent depressive disorder
Z91.82	Personal history of military deployment
Z91.49	Personal history of psychological trauma
F07.0	Personality change due to another medical condition
F12.921	Pharmaceutical cannabis receptor agonist–induced delirium (pharmaceutical cannabis receptor agonist medication taken as prescribed)
Z60.0	Phase of life problem
	Phencyclidine-induced anxiety disorder
F16.180	With mild use disorder
F16.280	With moderate or severe use disorder
F16.980	Without use disorder
	Phencyclidine-induced bipolar and related disorder
F16.14	With mild use disorder

ICD-10-CM   Disorder, condition, or problem

F16.24	With moderate or severe use disorder
F16.94	Without use disorder
	Phencyclidine-induced depressive disorder
F16.14	With mild use disorder
F16.24	With moderate or severe use disorder
F16.94	Without use disorder
	Phencyclidine-induced psychotic disorder
F16.159	With mild use disorder
F16.259	With moderate or severe use disorder
F16.959	Without use disorder
	Phencyclidine intoxication
F16.120	With mild use disorder
F16.220	With moderate or severe use disorder
F16.920	Without use disorder
	Phencyclidine intoxication delirium
F16.121	With mild use disorder
F16.221	With moderate or severe use disorder
F16.921	Without use disorder
	Phencyclidine use disorder
F16.10	Mild
F16.11	In early remission
F16.11	In sustained remission
F16.20	Moderate
F16.21	In early remission
F16.21	In sustained remission
F16.20	Severe
F16.21	In early remission

ICD-10-CM	Disorder, condition, or problem
F16.21	In sustained remission
	Pica
F50.89	In adults
F98.3	In children
F43.10	Posttraumatic stress disorder
F52.4	Premature (early) ejaculation
F32.81	Premenstrual dysphoric disorder
Z56.82	Problem related to current military deployment status
Z72.9	Problem related to lifestyle
Z60.2	Problem related to living alone
Z59.3	Problem related to living in a residential institution
Z55.8	Problems related to inadequate teaching
Z64.1	Problems related to multiparity
Z65.3	Problems related to other legal circumstances
Z65.2	Problems related to release from prison
Z64.0	Problems related to unwanted pregnancy
F43.81	Prolonged grief disorder
F95.0	Provisional tic disorder
F54	Psychological factors affecting other medical conditions
	Psychotic disorder due to another medical condition
F06.2	With delusions
F06.0	With hallucinations
F63.1	Pyromania
G47.52	Rapid eye movement sleep behavior disorder
F94.1	Reactive attachment disorder

ICD-10-CM	Disorder, condition, or problem
Z63.0	Relationship distress with spouse or intimate partner
Z65.8	Religious or spiritual problem
G25.81	Restless legs syndrome
F98.21	Rumination disorder
	Schizoaffective disorder
F25.0	Bipolar type
F25.1	Depressive type
F60.1	Schizoid personality disorder
F20.9	Schizophrenia
F20.81	Schizophreniform disorder
F21	Schizotypal personality disorder
Z55.1	Schooling unavailable and unattainable
	Sedative-, hypnotic-, or anxiolytic-induced anxiety disorder
F13.180	With mild use disorder
F13.280	With moderate or severe use disorder
F13.980	Without use disorder
	Sedative-, hypnotic-, or anxiolytic-induced bipolar and related disorder
F13.14	With mild use disorder
F13.24	With moderate or severe use disorder
F13.94	Without use disorder
F13.921	Sedative-, hypnotic-, or anxiolytic-induced delirium (sedative, hypnotic, or anxiolytic medication taken as prescribed)
F13.931	Sedative, hypnotic, or anxiolytic–induced delirium (during withdrawal from sedative, hypnotic, or anxiolytic medication taken as prescribed)

ICD-10-CM	Disorder, condition, or problem
	Sedative-, hypnotic-, or anxiolytic-induced depressive disorder
F13.14	With mild use disorder
F13.24	With moderate or severe use disorder
F13.94	Without use disorder
	Sedative-, hypnotic-, or anxiolytic-induced major neurocognitive disorder
F13.27	With moderate or severe use disorder
F13.97	Without use disorder
	Sedative-, hypnotic-, or anxiolytic-induced mild neurocognitive disorder
F13.188	With mild use disorder
F13.288	With moderate or severe use disorder
F13.988	Without use disorder
	Sedative-, hypnotic-, or anxiolytic-induced psychotic disorder
F13.159	With mild use disorder
F13.259	With moderate or severe use disorder
F13.959	Without use disorder
	Sedative-, hypnotic-, or anxiolytic-induced sexual dysfunction
F13.181	With mild use disorder
F13.281	With moderate or severe use disorder
F13.981	Without use disorder
	Sedative-, hypnotic-, or anxiolytic-induced sleep disorder
F13.182	With mild use disorder
F13.282	With moderate or severe use disorder
F13.982	Without use disorder

ICD-10-CM	Disorder, condition, or problem
	Sedative, hypnotic, or anxiolytic intoxication
F13.120	With mild use disorder
F13.220	With moderate or severe use disorder
F13.920	Without use disorder
	Sedative, hypnotic, or anxiolytic intoxication delirium
F13.121	With mild use disorder
F13.221	With moderate or severe use disorder
F13.921	Without use disorder
	Sedative, hypnotic, or anxiolytic use disorder
F13.10	Mild
F13.11	In early remission
F13.11	In sustained remission
F13.20	Moderate
F13.21	In early remission
F13.21	In sustained remission
F13.20	Severe
F13.21	In early remission
F13.21	In sustained remission
	Sedative, hypnotic, or anxiolytic withdrawal, With perceptual disturbances
F13.132	With mild use disorder
F13.232	With moderate or severe use disorder
F13.932	Without use disorder
	Sedative, hypnotic, or anxiolytic withdrawal, Without perceptual disturbances
F13.130	With mild use disorder
F13.230	With moderate or severe use disorder
F13.930	Without use disorder

ICD-10-CM	Disorder, condition, or problem
	Sedative, hypnotic, or anxiolytic withdrawal delirium
F13.131	With mild use disorder
F13.231	With moderate or severe use disorder
F13.931	Without use disorder
F94.0	Selective mutism
F93.0	Separation anxiety disorder
Z70.9	Sex counseling
Z56.81	Sexual harassment on the job
F65.51	Sexual masochism disorder
F65.52	Sexual sadism disorder
Z62.891	Sibling relational problem
	Sleep-related hypoventilation
G47.36	Comorbid sleep-related hypoventilation
G47.35	Congenital central alveolar hypoventilation
G47.34	Idiopathic hypoventilation
F40.10	Social anxiety disorder
Z60.4	Social exclusion or rejection
F80.82	Social (pragmatic) communication disorder
F45.1	Somatic symptom disorder
	Specific learning disorder
F81.2	With impairment in mathematics
F81.0	With impairment in reading
F81.81	With impairment in written expression
	Specific phobia
F40.218	Animal
	Blood-injection-injury
F40.230	Fear of blood

ICD-10-CM   Disorder, condition, or problem

F40.231	Fear of injections and transfusions
F40.233	Fear of injury
F40.232	Fear of other medical care
F40.228	Natural environment
F40.298	Other
F40.248	Situational
F80.0	Speech sound disorder
	Spouse or partner abuse, Psychological, Confirmed
T74.31XA	Initial encounter
T74.31XD	Subsequent encounter
	Spouse or partner abuse, Psychological, Suspected
T76.31XA	Initial encounter
T76.31XD	Subsequent encounter
	Spouse or partner neglect, Confirmed
T74.01XA	Initial encounter
T74.01XD	Subsequent encounter
	Spouse or partner neglect, Suspected
T76.01XA	Initial encounter
T76.01XD	Subsequent encounter
	Spouse or partner violence, Physical, Confirmed
T74.11XA	Initial encounter
T74.11XD	Subsequent encounter
	Spouse or partner violence, Physical, Suspected
T76.11XA	Initial encounter
T76.11XD	Subsequent encounter
	Spouse or partner violence, Sexual, Confirmed
T74.21XA	Initial encounter

ICD-10-CM Disorder, condition, or problem

T74.21XD	Subsequent encounter
	Spouse or partner violence, Sexual, Suspected
T76.21XA	Initial encounter
T76.21XD	Subsequent encounter
F98.4	Stereotypic movement disorder
	Stimulant intoxication *(see amphetamine-type substance, cocaine, or other or unspecified stimulant intoxication for specific codes)*
	Stimulant use disorder *(see amphetamine-type substance, cocaine, or other or unspecified stimulant use disorder for specific codes)*
	Stimulant withdrawal *(see amphetamine-type substance, cocaine, or other or unspecified stimulant withdrawal for specific codes)*
Z56.3	Stressful work schedule
F80.81	Stuttering (childhood-onset fluency disorder)
	Substance intoxication delirium *(see specific substances for codes)*
	Substance withdrawal delirium *(see specific substances for codes)*
	Substance/medication-induced anxiety disorder *(see specific substances for codes)*
	Substance/medication-induced bipolar and related disorder *(see specific substances for codes)*
	Substance/medication-induced depressive disorder *(see specific substances for codes)*
	Substance/medication-induced major or mild neurocognitive disorder *(see specific substances for codes)*
	Substance/medication-induced obsessive-compulsive and related disorder *(see specific substances for codes)*

ICD-10-CM Disorder, condition, or problem

	Substance/medication-induced psychotic disorder (*see specific substances for codes*)
	Substance/medication-induced sexual dysfunction (*see specific substances for codes*)
	Substance/medication-induced sleep disorder (*see specific substances for codes*)
	Suicidal behavior, current
T14.91XA	Initial encounter
T14.91XD	Subsequent encounter
Z91.51	Suicidal behavior, history of
G25.71	Tardive akathisia
G24.01	Tardive dyskinesia
G24.09	Tardive dystonia
Z60.5	Target of (perceived) adverse discrimination or persecution
Z56.2	Threat of job loss
	Tic disorders
F95.8	Other specified tic disorder
F95.1	Persistent (chronic) motor or vocal tic disorder
F95.0	Provisional tic disorder
F95.2	Tourette's disorder
F95.9	Unspecified tic disorder
F17.208	Tobacco-induced sleep disorder, With moderate or severe use disorder
	Tobacco use disorder
Z72.0	Mild
F17.200	Moderate
F17.201	In early remission
F17.201	In sustained remission

ICD-10-CM   Disorder, condition, or problem

F17.200	Severe
F17.201	In early remission
F17.201	In sustained remission
F17.203	Tobacco withdrawal
F95.2	Tourette's disorder
F65.1	Transvestic disorder
F63.3	Trichotillomania (hair-pulling disorder)
Z75.3	Unavailability or inaccessibility of health care facilities
Z75.4	Unavailability or inaccessibility of other helping agencies
Z63.4	Uncomplicated bereavement
Z56.5	Uncongenial work environment
Z55.3	Underachievement in school
Z56.0	Unemployment
F10.99	Unspecified alcohol-related disorder
F41.9	Unspecified anxiety disorder
F90.9	Unspecified attention-deficit/hyperactivity disorder
F31.9	Unspecified bipolar and related disorder
F15.99	Unspecified caffeine-related disorder
F12.99	Unspecified cannabis-related disorder
F06.1	Unspecified catatonia (*code first* R29.818 other symptoms involving nervous and musculoskeletal systems)
F80.9	Unspecified communication disorder
F05	Unspecified delirium
F32.A	Unspecified depressive disorder
F91.9	Unspecified disruptive, impulse-control, and conduct disorder

ICD-10-CM	Disorder, condition, or problem
F44.9	Unspecified dissociative disorder
	Unspecified elimination disorder
R15.9	With fecal symptoms
R32	With urinary symptoms
F50.9	Unspecified feeding or eating disorder
F64.9	Unspecified gender dysphoria
F16.99	Unspecified hallucinogen-related disorder
G47.10	Unspecified hypersomnolence disorder
F18.99	Unspecified inhalant-related disorder
G47.00	Unspecified insomnia disorder
F79	Unspecified intellectual developmental disorder (intellectual disability)
F99	Unspecified mental disorder
F09	Unspecified mental disorder due to another medical condition
F39	Unspecified mood disorder
R41.9	Unspecified neurocognitive disorder
F89	Unspecified neurodevelopmental disorder
F42.9	Unspecified obsessive-compulsive and related disorder
F11.99	Unspecified opioid-related disorder
F19.99	Unspecified other (or unknown) substance–related disorder
F65.9	Unspecified paraphilic disorder
F60.9	Unspecified personality disorder
F16.99	Unspecified phencyclidine-related disorder
F29	Unspecified schizophrenia spectrum and other psychotic disorder

ICD-10-CM	Disorder, condition, or problem
F13.99	Unspecified sedative-, hypnotic-, or anxiolytic-related disorder
F52.9	Unspecified sexual dysfunction
G47.9	Unspecified sleep-wake disorder
F45.9	Unspecified somatic symptom and related disorder
	Unspecified stimulant-related disorder
F15.99	Unspecified amphetamine-type substance–related disorder
F14.99	Unspecified cocaine-related disorder
F15.99	Unspecified other stimulant–related disorder
F95.9	Unspecified tic disorder
F17.209	Unspecified tobacco-related disorder
F43.9	Unspecified trauma- and stressor-related disorder
Z62.29	Upbringing away from parents
Z65.4	Victim of crime
Z65.4	Victim of terrorism or torture
F65.3	Voyeuristic disorder
Z91.83	Wandering associated with a mental disorder

For periodic DSM-5-TR coding and other updates, see www.dsm5.org.

ICD-10-CM	Disorder, condition, or problem
E66.9	Overweight or obesity
F01.50	Major neurocognitive disorder probably due to vascular disease, Unspecified severity, Without accompanying behavioral or psychological disturbance *(no additional medical code)*
F01.511	Major neurocognitive disorder probably due to vascular disease, Unspecified severity, With agitation *(no additional medical code)*
F01.518	Major neurocognitive disorder probably due to vascular disease, Unspecified severity, With other behavioral or psychological disturbance *(no additional medical code)*
F01.52	Major neurocognitive disorder probably due to vascular disease, Unspecified severity, With psychotic disturbance *(no additional medical code)*
F01.53	Major neurocognitive disorder probably due to vascular disease, Unspecified severity, With mood symptoms *(no additional medical code)*
F01.54	Major neurocognitive disorder probably due to vascular disease, Unspecified severity, With anxiety *(no additional medical code)*
F01.A0	Major neurocognitive disorder probably due to vascular disease, Mild, Without accompanying behavioral or psychological disturbance *(no additional medical code)*

ICD-10-CM   **Disorder, condition, or problem**

F01.A11	Major neurocognitive disorder probably due to vascular disease, Mild, With agitation *(no additional medical code)*
F01.A18	Major neurocognitive disorder probably due to vascular disease, Mild, With other behavioral or psychological disturbance *(no additional medical code)*
F01.A2	Major neurocognitive disorder probably due to vascular disease, Mild, With psychotic disturbance *(no additional medical code)*
F01.A3	Major neurocognitive disorder probably due to vascular disease, Mild, With mood symptoms *(no additional medical code)*
F01.A4	Major neurocognitive disorder probably due to vascular disease, Mild, With anxiety *(no additional medical code)*
F01.B0	Major neurocognitive disorder probably due to vascular disease, Moderate, Without accompanying behavioral or psychological disturbance *(no additional medical code)*
F01.B11	Major neurocognitive disorder probably due to vascular disease, Moderate, With agitation *(no additional medical code)*
F01.B18	Major neurocognitive disorder probably due to vascular disease, Moderate, With other behavioral or psychological disturbance *(no additional medical code)*
F01.B2	Major neurocognitive disorder probably due to vascular disease, Moderate, With psychotic disturbance *(no additional medical code)*
F01.B3	Major neurocognitive disorder probably due to vascular disease, Moderate, With mood symptoms *(no additional medical code)*

ICD-10-CM Disorder, condition, or problem

F01.B4   Major neurocognitive disorder probably due to
          vascular disease, Moderate, With anxiety
          (no additional medical code)

F01.C0   Major neurocognitive disorder probably due to
          vascular disease, Severe, Without accompanying
          behavioral or psychological disturbance
          (no additional medical code)

F01.C11   Major neurocognitive disorder probably due to
          vascular disease, Severe, With agitation *(no
          additional medical code)*

F01.C18   Major neurocognitive disorder probably due to
          vascular disease, Severe, With other behavioral or
          psychological disturbance *(no additional medical code)*

F01.C2   Major neurocognitive disorder probably due to
          vascular disease, Severe, With psychotic
          disturbance *(no additional medical code)*

F01.C3   Major neurocognitive disorder probably due to
          vascular disease, Severe, With mood symptoms
          (no additional medical code)

F01.C4   Major neurocognitive disorder probably due to
          vascular disease, Severe, With anxiety *(no additional
          medical code)*

F02.80   Major neurocognitive disorder due to another
          medical condition, Unspecified severity, Without
          accompanying behavioral or psychological
          disturbance *(code first* the other medical condition)

F02.80   Major neurocognitive disorder due to HIV
          infection, Unspecified severity, Without
          accompanying behavioral or psychological
          disturbance *(code first* B20 HIV infection)

ICD-10-CM   Disorder, condition, or problem

F02.80	Major neurocognitive disorder due to Huntington's disease, Unspecified severity, Without accompanying behavioral or psychological disturbance (*code first* G10 Huntington's disease)
F02.80	Major neurocognitive disorder due to multiple etiologies, Unspecified severity, Without accompanying behavioral or psychological disturbance (*code first* the other medical etiologies)
F02.80	Major neurocognitive disorder due to prion disease, Unspecified severity, Without accompanying behavioral or psychological disturbance (*code first* A81.9 prion disease)
F02.80	Major neurocognitive disorder due to probable Alzheimer's disease, Unspecified severity, Without accompanying behavioral or psychological disturbance (*code first* G30.9 Alzheimer's disease)
F02.80	Major neurocognitive disorder due to probable frontotemporal degeneration, Unspecified severity, Without accompanying behavioral or psychological disturbance (*code first* G31.09 frontotemporal degeneration)
F02.80	Major neurocognitive disorder with probable Lewy bodies, Unspecified severity, Without accompanying behavioral or psychological disturbance (*code first* G31.83 Lewy body disease)
F02.80	Major neurocognitive disorder probably due to Parkinson's disease, Unspecified severity, Without accompanying behavioral or psychological disturbance (*code first* G20.C Parkinson's disease)

ICD-10-CM Disorder, condition, or problem

F02.80	Major neurocognitive disorder due to traumatic brain injury, Unspecified severity, Without accompanying behavioral or psychological disturbance (*code first* S06.2XAS diffuse traumatic brain injury with loss of consciousness of unspecified duration, sequela)
F02.811	Major neurocognitive disorder due to another medical condition, Unspecified severity, With agitation (*code first* the other medical condition)
F02.811	Major neurocognitive disorder due to HIV infection, Unspecified severity, With agitation (*code first* B20 HIV infection)
F02.811	Major neurocognitive disorder due to Huntington's disease, Unspecified severity, With agitation (*code first* G10 Huntington's disease)
F02.811	Major neurocognitive disorder due to multiple etiologies, Unspecified severity, With agitation (*code first* the other medical etiologies)
F02.811	Major neurocognitive disorder due to prion disease, Unspecified severity, With agitation (*code first* A81.9 prion disease)
F02.811	Major neurocognitive disorder due to probable Alzheimer's disease, Unspecified severity, With agitation (*code first* G30.9 Alzheimer's disease)
F02.811	Major neurocognitive disorder due to probable frontotemporal degeneration, Unspecified severity, With agitation (*code first* G31.09 frontotemporal degeneration)
F02.811	Major neurocognitive disorder with probable Lewy bodies, Unspecified severity, With agitation (*code first* G31.83 Lewy body disease)

ICD-10-CM   Disorder, condition, or problem

F02.811   Major neurocognitive disorder probably due to Parkinson's disease, Unspecified severity, With agitation (*code first* G20.C Parkinson's disease)

F02.811   Major neurocognitive disorder due to traumatic brain injury, Unspecified severity, With agitation (*code first* S06.2XAS diffuse traumatic brain injury with loss of consciousness of unspecified duration, sequela)

F02.818   Major neurocognitive disorder due to another medical condition, Unspecified severity, With other behavioral or psychological disturbance (*code first* the other medical condition)

F02.818   Major neurocognitive disorder due to HIV infection, Unspecified severity, With other behavioral or psychological disturbance (*code first* B20 HIV infection)

F02.818   Major neurocognitive disorder due to Huntington's disease, Unspecified severity, With other behavioral or psychological disturbance (*code first* G10 Huntington's disease)

F02.818   Major neurocognitive disorder due to multiple etiologies, Unspecified severity, With other behavioral or psychological disturbance (*code first* the other medical etiologies)

F02.818   Major neurocognitive disorder due to prion disease, Unspecified severity, With other behavioral or psychological disturbance (*code first* A81.9 prion disease)

F02.818   Major neurocognitive disorder due to probable Alzheimer's disease, Unspecified severity, With other behavioral or psychological disturbance (*code first* G30.9 Alzheimer's disease)

ICD-10-CM   Disorder, condition, or problem

F02.818	Major neurocognitive disorder due to probable frontotemporal degeneration, Unspecified severity, With other behavioral or psychological disturbance (*code first* G31.09 frontotemporal degeneration)
F02.818	Major neurocognitive disorder with probable Lewy bodies, Unspecified severity, With other behavioral or psychological disturbance (*code first* G31.83 Lewy body disease)
F02.818	Major neurocognitive disorder probably due to Parkinson's disease, Unspecified severity, With other behavioral or psychological disturbance (*code first* G20.C Parkinson's disease)
F02.818	Major neurocognitive disorder due to traumatic brain injury, Unspecified severity, With other behavioral or psychological disturbance (*code first* S06.2XAS diffuse traumatic brain injury with loss of consciousness of unspecified duration, sequela)
F02.82	Major neurocognitive disorder due to another medical condition, Unspecified severity, With psychotic disturbance (*code first* the other medical condition
F02.82	Major neurocognitive disorder due to HIV infection, Unspecified severity, With psychotic disturbance (*code first* B20 HIV infection)
F02.82	Major neurocognitive disorder due to Huntington's disease, Unspecified severity, With psychotic disturbance (*code first* G10 Huntington's disease)
F02.82	Major neurocognitive disorder due to multiple etiologies, Unspecified severity, With psychotic disturbance (*code first* the other medical etiologies)

ICD-10-CM Disorder, condition, or problem

F02.82	Major neurocognitive disorder due to prion disease, Unspecified severity, With psychotic disturbance (*code first* A81.9 prion disease)
F02.82	Major neurocognitive disorder due to probable Alzheimer's disease, Unspecified severity, With psychotic disturbance (*code first* G30.9 Alzheimer's disease)
F02.82	Major neurocognitive disorder due to probable frontotemporal degeneration, Unspecified severity, With psychotic disturbance (*code first* G31.09 frontotemporal degeneration)
F02.82	Major neurocognitive disorder with probable Lewy bodies, Unspecified severity, With psychotic disturbance (*code first* G31.83 Lewy body disease)
F02.82	Major neurocognitive disorder probably due to Parkinson's disease, Unspecified severity, With psychotic disturbance (*code first* G20.C Parkinson's disease)
F02.82	Major neurocognitive disorder due to traumatic brain injury, Unspecified severity, With psychotic disturbance (*code first* S06.2XAS diffuse traumatic brain injury with loss of consciousness of unspecified duration, sequela)
F02.83	Major neurocognitive disorder due to another medical condition, Unspecified severity, With mood symptoms (*code first* the other medical condition)
F02.83	Major neurocognitive disorder due to HIV infection, Unspecified severity, With mood symptoms (*code first* B20 HIV infection)
F02.83	Major neurocognitive disorder due to Huntington's disease, Unspecified severity, With mood symptoms (*code first* G10 Huntington's disease)

ICD-10-CM	Disorder, condition, or problem
F02.83	Major neurocognitive disorder due to multiple etiologies, Unspecified severity, With mood symptoms (*code first* the other medical etiologies)
F02.83	Major neurocognitive disorder due to prion disease, Unspecified severity, With mood symptoms (*code first* A81.9 prion disease)
F02.83	Major neurocognitive disorder due to probable Alzheimer's disease, Unspecified severity, With mood symptoms (*code first* G30.9 Alzheimer's disease)
F02.83	Major neurocognitive disorder due to probable frontotemporal degeneration, Unspecified severity, With mood symptoms (*code first* G31.09 frontotemporal degeneration)
F02.83	Major neurocognitive disorder with probable Lewy bodies, Unspecified severity, With mood symptoms (*code first* G31.83 Lewy body disease)
F02.83	Major neurocognitive disorder probably due to Parkinson's disease, Unspecified severity, With mood symptoms (*code first* G20.C Parkinson's disease)
F02.83	Major neurocognitive disorder due to traumatic brain injury, Unspecified severity, With mood symptoms (*code first* S06.2XAS diffuse traumatic brain injury with loss of consciousness of unspecified duration, sequela)
F02.84	Major neurocognitive disorder due to another medical condition, Unspecified severity, With anxiety (*code first* the other medical condition)
F02.84	Major neurocognitive disorder due to HIV infection, Unspecified severity, With anxiety (*code first* B20 HIV infection)

ICD-10-CM	Disorder, condition, or problem
F02.84	Major neurocognitive disorder due to Huntington's disease, Unspecified severity, With anxiety (*code first* G10 Huntington's disease)
F02.84	Major neurocognitive disorder due to multiple etiologies, Unspecified severity, With anxiety (*code first* the other medical etiologies)
F02.84	Major neurocognitive disorder due to prion disease, Unspecified severity, With anxiety (*code first* A81.9 prion disease)
F02.84	Major neurocognitive disorder due to probable Alzheimer's disease, Unspecified severity, With anxiety (*code first* G30.9 Alzheimer's disease)
F02.84	Major neurocognitive disorder due to probable frontotemporal degeneration, Unspecified severity, With anxiety (*code first* G31.09 frontotemporal degeneration)
F02.84	Major neurocognitive disorder with probable Lewy bodies, Unspecified severity, With anxiety (*code first* G31.83 Lewy body disease)
F02.84	Major neurocognitive disorder probably due to Parkinson's disease, Unspecified severity, With anxiety (*code first* G20.C Parkinson's disease)
F02.84	Major neurocognitive disorder due to traumatic brain injury, Unspecified severity, With anxiety (*code first* S06.2XAS diffuse traumatic brain injury with loss of consciousness of unspecified duration, sequela)
F02.A0	Major neurocognitive disorder due to another medical condition, Mild, Without accompanying behavioral or psychological disturbance (*code first* the other medical condition)

ICD-10-CM Disorder, condition, or problem

F02.A0   Major neurocognitive disorder due to HIV infection, Mild, Without accompanying behavioral or psychological disturbance (*code first* B20 HIV infection)

F02.A0   Major neurocognitive disorder due to Huntington's disease, Mild, Without accompanying behavioral or psychological disturbance (*code first* G10 Huntington's disease)

F02.A0   Major neurocognitive disorder due to multiple etiologies, Mild, Without accompanying behavioral or psychological disturbance (*code first* the other medical etiologies)

F02.A0   Major neurocognitive disorder due to prion disease, Mild, Without accompanying behavioral or psychological disturbance (*code first* A81.9 prion disease)

F02.A0   Major neurocognitive disorder due to probable Alzheimer's disease, Mild, Without accompanying behavioral or psychological disturbance (*code first* G30.9 Alzheimer's disease)

F02.A0   Major neurocognitive disorder due to probable frontotemporal degeneration, Mild, Without accompanying behavioral or psychological disturbance (*code first* G31.09 frontotemporal degeneration)

F02.A0   Major neurocognitive disorder with probable Lewy bodies, Mild, Without accompanying behavioral or psychological disturbance (*code first* G31.83 Lewy body disease)

F02.A0   Major neurocognitive disorder probably due to Parkinson's disease, Mild, Without accompanying behavioral or psychological disturbance (*code first* G20.C Parkinson's disease)

ICD-10-CM	Disorder, condition, or problem
F02.A0	Major neurocognitive disorder due to traumatic brain injury, Mild, Without accompanying behavioral or psychological disturbance (*code first* S06.2XAS diffuse traumatic brain injury with loss of consciousness of unspecified duration, sequela)
F02.A11	Major neurocognitive disorder due to another medical condition, Mild, With agitation (*code first* the other medical condition)
F02.A11	Major neurocognitive disorder due to HIV infection, Mild, With agitation (*code first* B20 HIV infection)
F02.A11	Major neurocognitive disorder due to Huntington's disease, Mild, With agitation (*code first* G10 Huntington's disease)
F02.A11	Major neurocognitive disorder due to multiple etiologies, Mild, With agitation (*code first* the other medical etiologies)
F02.A11	Major neurocognitive disorder due to prion disease, Mild, With agitation (*code first* A81.9 prion disease)
F02.A11	Major neurocognitive disorder due to probable Alzheimer's disease, Mild, With agitation (*code first* G30.9 Alzheimer's disease)
F02.A11	Major neurocognitive disorder due to probable frontotemporal degeneration, Mild, With agitation (*code first* G31.09 frontotemporal degeneration)
F02.A11	Major neurocognitive disorder with probable Lewy bodies, Mild, With agitation (*code first* G31.83 Lewy body disease)
F02.A11	Major neurocognitive disorder probably due to Parkinson's disease, Mild, With agitation (*code first* G20.C Parkinson's disease)

ICD-10-CM Disorder, condition, or problem

F02.A11	Major neurocognitive disorder due to traumatic brain injury, Mild, With agitation (*code first* S06.2XAS diffuse traumatic brain injury with loss of consciousness of unspecified duration, sequela)
F02.A18	Major neurocognitive disorder due to another medical condition, Mild, With other behavioral or psychological disturbance (*code first* the other medical condition)
F02.A18	Major neurocognitive disorder due to HIV infection, Mild, With other behavioral or psychological disturbance (*code first* B20 HIV infection)
F02.A18	Major neurocognitive disorder due to Huntington's disease, Mild, With other behavioral or psychological disturbance (*code first* G10 Huntington's disease)
F02.A18	Major neurocognitive disorder due to multiple etiologies, Mild, With other behavioral or psychological disturbance (*code first* the other medical etiologies)
F02.A18	Major neurocognitive disorder due to prion disease, Mild, With other behavioral or psychological disturbance (*code first* A81.9 prion disease)
F02.A18	Major neurocognitive disorder due to probable Alzheimer's disease, Mild, With other behavioral or psychological disturbance (*code first* G30.9 Alzheimer's disease)
F02.A18	Major neurocognitive disorder due to probable frontotemporal degeneration, Mild, With other behavioral or psychological disturbance (*code first* G31.09 frontotemporal degeneration)

ICD-10-CM Disorder, condition, or problem

F02.A18	Major neurocognitive disorder with probable Lewy bodies, Mild, With other behavioral or psychological disturbance (*code first* G31.83 Lewy body disease)
F02.A18	Major neurocognitive disorder probably due to Parkinson's disease, Mild, With other behavioral or psychological disturbance (*code first* G20.C Parkinson's disease)
F02.A18	Major neurocognitive disorder due to traumatic brain injury, Mild, With other behavioral or psychological disturbance (*code first* S06.2XAS diffuse traumatic brain injury with loss of consciousness of unspecified duration, sequela)
F02.A2	Major neurocognitive disorder due to another medical condition, Mild, With psychotic disturbance (*code first* the other medical condition)
F02.A2	Major neurocognitive disorder due to HIV infection, Mild, With psychotic disturbance (*code first* B20 HIV infection)
F02.A2	Major neurocognitive disorder due to Huntington's disease, Mild, With psychotic disturbance (*code first* G10 Huntington's disease)
F02.A2	Major neurocognitive disorder due to multiple etiologies, Mild, With psychotic disturbance (*code first* the other medical etiologies)
F02.A2	Major neurocognitive disorder due to prion disease, Mild, With psychotic disturbance (*code first* A81.9 prion disease)
F02.A2	Major neurocognitive disorder due to probable Alzheimer's disease, Mild, With psychotic disturbance (*code first* G30.9 Alzheimer's disease)

ICD-10-CM	Disorder, condition, or problem
F02.A2	Major neurocognitive disorder due to probable frontotemporal degeneration, Mild, With psychotic disturbance (*code first* G31.09 frontotemporal degeneration)
F02.A2	Major neurocognitive disorder with probable Lewy bodies, Mild, With psychotic disturbance (*code first* G31.83 Lewy body disease)
F02.A2	Major neurocognitive disorder probably due to Parkinson's disease, Mild, With psychotic disturbance (*code first* G20.C Parkinson's disease)
F02.A2	Major neurocognitive disorder due to traumatic brain injury, Mild, With psychotic disturbance (*code first* S06.2XAS diffuse traumatic brain injury with loss of consciousness of unspecified duration, sequela)
F02.A3	Major neurocognitive disorder due to another medical condition, Mild, With mood symptoms (*code first* the other medical condition)
F02.A3	Major neurocognitive disorder due to HIV infection, Mild, With mood symptoms (*code first* B20 HIV infection)
F02.A3	Major neurocognitive disorder due to Huntington's disease, Mild, With mood symptoms (*code first* G10 Huntington's disease)
F02.A3	Major neurocognitive disorder due to multiple etiologies, Mild, With mood symptoms (*code first* the other medical etiologies)
F02.A3	Major neurocognitive disorder due to prion disease, Mild, With mood symptoms (*code first* A81.9 prion disease)
F02.A3	Major neurocognitive disorder due to probable Alzheimer's disease, Mild, With mood symptoms (*code first* G30.9 Alzheimer's disease)

ICD-10-CM	Disorder, condition, or problem
F02.A3	Major neurocognitive disorder due to probable frontotemporal degeneration, Mild, With mood symptoms (*code first* G31.09 frontotemporal degeneration)
F02.A3	Major neurocognitive disorder with probable Lewy bodies, Mild, With mood symptoms (*code first* G31.83 Lewy body disease)
F02.A3	Major neurocognitive disorder probably due to Parkinson's disease, Mild, With mood symptoms (*code first* G20.C Parkinson's disease)
F02.A3	Major neurocognitive disorder due to traumatic brain injury, Mild, With mood symptoms (*code first* S06.2XAS diffuse traumatic brain injury with loss of consciousness of unspecified duration, sequela)
F02.A4	Major neurocognitive disorder due to another medical condition, Mild, With anxiety (*code first* the other medical condition
F02.A4	Major neurocognitive disorder due to HIV infection, Mild, With anxiety (*code first* B20 HIV infection)
F02.A4	Major neurocognitive disorder due to Huntington's disease, Mild, With anxiety (*code first* G10 Huntington's disease)
F02.A4	Major neurocognitive disorder due to multiple etiologies, Mild, With anxiety (*code first* the other medical etiologies)
F02.A4	Major neurocognitive disorder due to prion disease, Mild, With anxiety (*code first* A81.9 prion disease)
F02.A4	Major neurocognitive disorder due to probable Alzheimer's disease, Mild, With anxiety (*code first* G30.9 Alzheimer's disease)

ICD-10-CM Disorder, condition, or problem

F02.A4 — Major neurocognitive disorder due to probable frontotemporal degeneration, Mild, With anxiety (*code first* G31.09 frontotemporal degeneration)

F02.A4 — Major neurocognitive disorder with probable Lewy bodies, Mild, With anxiety (*code first* G31.83 Lewy body disease)

F02.A4 — Major neurocognitive disorder probably due to Parkinson's disease, Mild, With anxiety (*code first* G20.C Parkinson's disease)

F02.A4 — Major neurocognitive disorder due to traumatic brain injury, Mild, With anxiety (*code first* S06.2XAS diffuse traumatic brain injury with loss of consciousness of unspecified duration, sequela)

F02.B0 — Major neurocognitive disorder due to another medical condition, Moderate, Without accompanying behavioral or psychological disturbance (*code first* the other medical condition)

F02.B0 — Major neurocognitive disorder due to HIV infection, Moderate, Without accompanying behavioral or psychological disturbance (*code first* B20 HIV infection)

F02.B0 — Major neurocognitive disorder due to Huntington's disease, Moderate, Without accompanying behavioral or psychological disturbance (*code first* G10 Huntington's disease)

F02.B0 — Major neurocognitive disorder due to multiple etiologies, Moderate, Without accompanying behavioral or psychological disturbance (*code first* the other medical etiologies)

F02.B0 — Major neurocognitive disorder due to prion disease, Moderate, Without accompanying behavioral or psychological disturbance (*code first* A81.9 prion disease)

ICD-10-CM	Disorder, condition, or problem
F02.B0	Major neurocognitive disorder due to probable Alzheimer's disease, Moderate, Without accompanying behavioral or psychological disturbance (*code first* G30.9 Alzheimer's disease)
F02.B0	Major neurocognitive disorder due to probable frontotemporal degeneration, Moderate, Without accompanying behavioral or psychological disturbance (*code first* G31.09 frontotemporal degeneration)
F02.B0	Major neurocognitive disorder with probable Lewy bodies, Moderate, Without accompanying behavioral or psychological disturbance (*code first* G31.83 Lewy body disease)
F02.B0	Major neurocognitive disorder probably due to Parkinson's disease, Moderate, Without accompanying behavioral or psychological disturbance (*code first* G20.C Parkinson's disease)
F02.B0	Major neurocognitive disorder due to traumatic brain injury, Moderate, Without accompanying behavioral or psychological disturbance (*code first* S06.2XAS diffuse traumatic brain injury with loss of consciousness of unspecified duration, sequela)
F02.B11	Major neurocognitive disorder due to another medical condition, Moderate, With agitation (*code first* the other medical condition)
F02.B11	Major neurocognitive disorder due to HIV infection, Moderate, With agitation (*code first* B20 HIV infection)
F02.B11	Major neurocognitive disorder due to Huntington's disease, Moderate, With agitation (*code first* G10 Huntington's disease)

ICD-10-CM   Disorder, condition, or problem

F02.B11	Major neurocognitive disorder due to multiple etiologies, Moderate, With agitation (*code first* the other medical etiologies)
F02.B11	Major neurocognitive disorder due to prion disease, Moderate, With agitation (*code first* A81.9 prion disease)
F02.B11	Major neurocognitive disorder due to probable Alzheimer's disease, Moderate, With agitation (*code first* G30.9 Alzheimer's disease)
F02.B11	Major neurocognitive disorder due to probable frontotemporal degeneration, Moderate, With agitation (*code first* G31.09 frontotemporal degeneration)
F02.B11	Major neurocognitive disorder with probable Lewy bodies, Moderate, With agitation (*code first* G31.83 Lewy body disease)
F02.B11	Major neurocognitive disorder probably due to Parkinson's disease, Moderate, With agitation (*code first* G20.C Parkinson's disease)
F02.B11	Major neurocognitive disorder due to traumatic brain injury, Moderate, With agitation (*code first* S06.2XAS diffuse traumatic brain injury with loss of consciousness of unspecified duration, sequela)
F02.B18	Major neurocognitive disorder due to another medical condition, Moderate, With other behavioral or psychological disturbance (*code first* the other medical condition)
F02.B18	Major neurocognitive disorder due to HIV infection, Moderate, With other behavioral or psychological disturbance (*code first* B20 HIV infection)

ICD-10-CM	Disorder, condition, or problem
F02.B18	Major neurocognitive disorder due to Huntington's disease, Moderate, With other behavioral or psychological disturbance (*code first* G10 Huntington's disease)
F02.B18	Major neurocognitive disorder due to multiple etiologies, Moderate, With other behavioral or psychological disturbance (*code first* the other medical etiologies)
F02.B18	Major neurocognitive disorder due to prion disease, Moderate, With other behavioral or psychological disturbance (*code first* A81.9 prion disease)
F02.B18	Major neurocognitive disorder due to probable Alzheimer's disease, Moderate, With other behavioral or psychological disturbance (*code first* G30.9 Alzheimer's disease)
F02.B18	Major neurocognitive disorder due to probable frontotemporal degeneration, Moderate, With other behavioral or psychological disturbance (*code first* G31.09 frontotemporal degeneration)
F02.B18	Major neurocognitive disorder with probable Lewy bodies, Moderate, With other behavioral or psychological disturbance (*code first* G31.83 Lewy body disease)
F02.B18	Major neurocognitive disorder probably due to Parkinson's disease, Moderate, With other behavioral or psychological disturbance (*code first* G20.C Parkinson's disease)
F02.B18	Major neurocognitive disorder due to traumatic brain injury, Moderate, With other behavioral or psychological disturbance (*code first* S06.2XAS diffuse traumatic brain injury with loss of consciousness of unspecified duration, sequela)

ICD-10-CM Disorder, condition, or problem

F02.B2	Major neurocognitive disorder due to another medical condition, Moderate, With psychotic disturbance (*code first* the other medical condition)
F02.B2	Major neurocognitive disorder due to HIV infection, Moderate, With psychotic disturbance (*code first* B20 HIV infection)
F02.B2	Major neurocognitive disorder due to Huntington's disease, Moderate, With psychotic disturbance (*code first* G10 Huntington's disease)
F02.B2	Major neurocognitive disorder due to multiple etiologies, Moderate, With psychotic disturbance (*code first* the other medical etiologies)
F02.B2	Major neurocognitive disorder due to prion disease, Moderate, With psychotic disturbance (*code first* A81.9 prion disease)
F02.B2	Major neurocognitive disorder due to probable Alzheimer's disease, Moderate, With psychotic disturbance (*code first* G30.9 Alzheimer's disease)
F02.B2	Major neurocognitive disorder due to probable frontotemporal degeneration, Moderate, With psychotic disturbance (*code first* G31.09 frontotemporal degeneration)
F02.B2	Major neurocognitive disorder with probable Lewy bodies, Moderate, With psychotic disturbance (*code first* G31.83 Lewy body disease)
F02.B2	Major neurocognitive disorder probably due to Parkinson's disease, Moderate, With psychotic disturbance (*code first* G20.C Parkinson's disease)
F02.B2	Major neurocognitive disorder due to traumatic brain injury, Moderate, With psychotic disturbance (*code first* S06.2XAS diffuse traumatic brain injury with loss of consciousness of unspecified duration, sequela)

ICD-10-CM	Disorder, condition, or problem
F02.B3	Major neurocognitive disorder due to another medical condition, Moderate, With mood symptoms (*code first* the other medical condition)
F02.B3	Major neurocognitive disorder due to HIV infection, Moderate, With mood symptoms (*code first* B20 HIV infection)
F02.B3	Major neurocognitive disorder due to Huntington's disease, Moderate, With mood symptoms (*code first* G10 Huntington's disease)
F02.B3	Major neurocognitive disorder due to multiple etiologies, Moderate, With mood symptoms (*code first* the other medical etiologies)
F02.B3	Major neurocognitive disorder due to prion disease, Moderate, With mood symptoms (*code first* A81.9 prion disease)
F02.B3	Major neurocognitive disorder due to probable Alzheimer's disease, Moderate, With mood symptoms (*code first* G30.9 Alzheimer's disease)
F02.B3	Major neurocognitive disorder due to probable frontotemporal degeneration, Moderate, With mood symptoms (*code first* G31.09 frontotemporal degeneration)
F02.B3	Major neurocognitive disorder with probable Lewy bodies, Moderate, With mood symptoms (*code first* G31.83 Lewy body disease)
F02.B3	Major neurocognitive disorder probably due to Parkinson's disease, Moderate, With mood symptoms (*code first* G20.C Parkinson's disease)
F02.B3	Major neurocognitive disorder due to traumatic brain injury, Moderate, With mood symptoms (*code first*s S06.2XAS diffuse traumatic brain injury with loss of consciousness of unspecified duration, sequela)

ICD-10-CM	Disorder, condition, or problem
F02.B4	Major neurocognitive disorder due to another medical condition, Moderate, With anxiety (*code first* the other medical condition)
F02.B4	Major neurocognitive disorder due to HIV infection, Moderate, With anxiety (*code first* B20 HIV infection)
F02.B4	Major neurocognitive disorder due to Huntington's disease, Moderate, With anxiety (*code first* G10 Huntington's disease)
F02.B4	Major neurocognitive disorder due to multiple etiologies, Moderate, With anxiety (*code first* the other medical etiologies)
F02.B4	Major neurocognitive disorder due to prion disease, Moderate, With anxiety (*code first* A81.9 prion disease)
F02.B4	Major neurocognitive disorder due to probable Alzheimer's disease, Moderate, With anxiety (*code first* G30.9 Alzheimer's disease)
F02.B4	Major neurocognitive disorder due to probable frontotemporal degeneration, Moderate, With anxiety (*code first* G31.09 frontotemporal degeneration)
F02.B4	Major neurocognitive disorder with probable Lewy bodies, Moderate, With anxiety (*code first* G31.83 Lewy body disease)
F02.B4	Major neurocognitive disorder probably due to Parkinson's disease, Moderate, With anxiety (*code first* G20.C Parkinson's disease)
F02.B4	Major neurocognitive disorder due to traumatic brain injury, Moderate, With anxiety (*code first* S06.2XAS diffuse traumatic brain injury with loss of consciousness of unspecified duration, sequela)

ICD-10-CM   Disorder, condition, or problem

F02.C0   Major neurocognitive disorder due to another medical condition, Severe, Without accompanying behavioral or psychological disturbance (*code first* the other medical condition)

F02.C0   Major neurocognitive disorder due to HIV infection, Severe, Without accompanying behavioral or psychological disturbance (*code first* B20 HIV infection)

F02.C0   Major neurocognitive disorder due to Huntington's disease, Severe, Without accompanying behavioral or psychological disturbance (*code first* G10 Huntington's disease)

F02.C0   Major neurocognitive disorder due to multiple etiologies, Severe, Without accompanying behavioral or psychological disturbance (*code first* the other medical etiologies)

F02.C0   Major neurocognitive disorder due to prion disease, Severe, Without accompanying behavioral or psychological disturbance (*code first* A81.9 prion disease)

F02.C0   Major neurocognitive disorder due to probable Alzheimer's disease, Severe, Without accompanying behavioral or psychological disturbance (*code first* G30.9 Alzheimer's disease)

F02.C0   Major neurocognitive disorder due to probable frontotemporal degeneration, Severe, Without accompanying behavioral or psychological disturbance (*code first* G31.09 frontotemporal degeneration)

F02.C0   Major neurocognitive disorder with probable Lewy bodies, Severe, Without accompanying behavioral or psychological disturbance (*code first* G31.83 Lewy body disease)

ICD-10-CM   Disorder, condition, or problem

F02.C0	Major neurocognitive disorder probably due to Parkinson's disease, Severe, Without accompanying behavioral or psychological disturbance (*code first* G20.C Parkinson's disease)
F02.C0	Major neurocognitive disorder due to traumatic brain injury, Severe, Without accompanying behavioral or psychological disturbance (*code first* S06.2XAS diffuse traumatic brain injury with loss of consciousness of unspecified duration, sequela)
F02.C11	Major neurocognitive disorder due to another medical condition, Severe, With agitation (*code first* the other medical condition)
F02.C11	Major neurocognitive disorder due to HIV infection, Severe, With agitation (*code first* B20 HIV infection)
F02.C11	Major neurocognitive disorder due to Huntington's disease, Severe, With agitation (*code first* G10 Huntington's disease)
F02.C11	Major neurocognitive disorder due to multiple etiologies, Severe, With agitation (*code first* the other medical etiologies)
F02.C11	Major neurocognitive disorder due to prion disease, Severe, With agitation (*code first* A81.9 prion disease)
F02.C11	Major neurocognitive disorder due to probable Alzheimer's disease, Severe, With agitation (*code first* G30.9 Alzheimer's disease)
F02.C11	Major neurocognitive disorder due to probable frontotemporal degeneration, Severe, With agitation (*code first* G31.09 frontotemporal degeneration)

ICD-10-CM Disorder, condition, or problem

F02.C11	Major neurocognitive disorder with probable Lewy bodies, Severe, With agitation (*code first* G31.83 Lewy body disease)
F02.C11	Major neurocognitive disorder probably due to Parkinson's disease, Severe, With agitation (*code first* G20.C Parkinson's disease)
F02.C11	Major neurocognitive disorder due to traumatic brain injury, Severe, With agitation (*code first* S06.2XAS diffuse traumatic brain injury with loss of consciousness of unspecified duration, sequela)
F02.C18	Major neurocognitive disorder due to another medical condition, Severe, With other behavioral or psychological disturbance (*code first* the other medical condition)
F02.C18	Major neurocognitive disorder due to HIV infection, Severe, With other behavioral or psychological disturbance (*code first* B20 HIV infection)
F02.C18	Major neurocognitive disorder due to Huntington's disease, Severe, With other behavioral or psychological disturbance (*code first* G10 Huntington's disease)
F02.C18	Major neurocognitive disorder due to multiple etiologies, Severe, With other behavioral or psychological disturbance (*code first* the other medical etiologies)
F02.C18	Major neurocognitive disorder due to prion disease, Severe, With other behavioral or psychological disturbance (*code first* A81.9 prion disease)
F02.C18	Major neurocognitive disorder due to probable Alzheimer's disease, Severe, With other behavioral or psychological disturbance (*code first* G30.9 Alzheimer's disease)

ICD-10-CM   Disorder, condition, or problem

F02.C18   Major neurocognitive disorder due to probable frontotemporal degeneration, Severe, With other behavioral or psychological disturbance (*code first* G31.09 frontotemporal degeneration)

F02.C18   Major neurocognitive disorder with probable Lewy bodies, Severe, With other behavioral or psychological disturbance (*code first* G31.83 Lewy body disease)

F02.C18   Major neurocognitive disorder probably due to Parkinson's disease, Severe, With other behavioral or psychological disturbance (*code first* G20.C Parkinson's disease)

F02.C18   Major neurocognitive disorder due to traumatic brain injury, Severe, With other behavioral or psychological disturbance (*code first* S06.2XAS diffuse traumatic brain injury with loss of consciousness of unspecified duration, sequela)

F02.C2   Major neurocognitive disorder due to another medical condition, Severe, With psychotic disturbance (*code first* the other medical condition)

F02.C2   Major neurocognitive disorder due to HIV infection, Severe, With psychotic disturbance (*code first* B20 HIV infection)

F02.C2   Major neurocognitive disorder due to Huntington's disease, Severe, With psychotic disturbance (*code first* G10 Huntington's disease)

F02.C2   Major neurocognitive disorder due to multiple etiologies, Severe, With psychotic disturbance (*code first* the other medical etiologies)

F02.C2   Major neurocognitive disorder due to prion disease, Severe, With psychotic disturbance (*code first* A81.9 prion disease)

ICD-10-CM	Disorder, condition, or problem
F02.C2	Major neurocognitive disorder due to probable Alzheimer's disease, Severe, With psychotic disturbance (*code first* G30.9 Alzheimer's disease)
F02.C2	Major neurocognitive disorder due to probable frontotemporal degeneration, Severe, With psychotic disturbance (*code first* G31.09 frontotemporal degeneration)
F02.C2	Major neurocognitive disorder with probable Lewy bodies, Severe, With psychotic disturbance (*code first* G31.83 Lewy body disease)
F02.C2	Major neurocognitive disorder probably due to Parkinson's disease, Severe, With psychotic disturbance (*code first* G20.C Parkinson's disease)
F02.C2	Major neurocognitive disorder due to traumatic brain injury, Severe, With psychotic disturbance (*code first* S06.2XAS diffuse traumatic brain injury with loss of consciousness of unspecified duration, sequela)
F02.C3	Major neurocognitive disorder due to another medical condition, Severe, With mood symptoms (*code first* the other medical condition)
F02.C3	Major neurocognitive disorder due to HIV infection, Severe, With mood symptoms (*code first* B20 HIV infection)
F02.C3	Major neurocognitive disorder due to Huntington's disease, Severe, With mood symptoms (*code first* G10 Huntington's disease)
F02.C3	Major neurocognitive disorder due to multiple etiologies, Severe, With mood symptoms (*code first* the other medical etiologies)
F02.C3	Major neurocognitive disorder due to prion disease, Severe, With mood symptoms (*code first* A81.9 prion disease)

ICD-10-CM	Disorder, condition, or problem
F02.C3	Major neurocognitive disorder due to probable Alzheimer's disease, Severe, With mood symptoms (*code first* G30.9 Alzheimer's disease)
F02.C3	Major neurocognitive disorder due to probable frontotemporal degeneration, Severe, With mood symptoms (*code first* G31.09 frontotemporal degeneration)
F02.C3	Major neurocognitive disorder with probable Lewy bodies, Severe, With mood symptoms (*code first* G31.83 Lewy body disease)
F02.C3	Major neurocognitive disorder probably due to Parkinson's disease, Severe, With mood symptoms (*code first* G20.C Parkinson's disease)
F02.C3	Major neurocognitive disorder due to traumatic brain injury, Severe, With mood symptoms (*code first* S06.2XAS diffuse traumatic brain injury with loss of consciousness of unspecified duration, sequela)
F02.C4	Major neurocognitive disorder due to another medical condition, Severe, With anxiety (*code first* the other medical condition)
F02.C4	Major neurocognitive disorder due to HIV infection, Severe, With anxiety (*code first* B20 HIV infection)
F02.C4	Major neurocognitive disorder due to Huntington's disease, Severe, With anxiety (*code first* G10 Huntington's disease)
F02.C4	Major neurocognitive disorder due to multiple etiologies, Severe, With anxiety (*code first* the other medical etiologies)
F02.C4	Major neurocognitive disorder due to prion disease, Severe, With anxiety (*code first* A81.9 prion disease)

ICD-10-CM   Disorder, condition, or problem

F02.C4	Major neurocognitive disorder due to probable Alzheimer's disease, Severe, With anxiety (*code first* G30.9 Alzheimer's disease)
F02.C4	Major neurocognitive disorder due to probable frontotemporal degeneration, Severe, With anxiety (*code first* G31.09 frontotemporal degeneration)
F02.C4	Major neurocognitive disorder with probable Lewy bodies, Severe, With anxiety (*code first* G31.83 Lewy body disease)
F02.C4	Major neurocognitive disorder probably due to Parkinson's disease, Severe, With anxiety (*code first* G20.C Parkinson's disease)
F02.C4	Major neurocognitive disorder due to traumatic brain injury, Severe, With anxiety (*code first* S06.2XAS diffuse traumatic brain injury with loss of consciousness of unspecified duration, sequela)
F03.90	Major neurocognitive disorder due to possible Alzheimer's disease, Unspecified severity, Without accompanying behavioral or psychological disturbance (*no additional medical code*)
F03.90	Major neurocognitive disorder due to possible frontotemporal degeneration, Unspecified severity, Without accompanying behavioral or psychological disturbance (*no additional medical code*)
F03.90	Major neurocognitive disorder with possible Lewy bodies, Unspecified severity, Without accompanying behavioral or psychological disturbance (*no additional medical code*)

ICD-10-CM Disorder, condition, or problem

F03.90	Major neurocognitive disorder possibly due to Parkinson's disease, Unspecified severity, Without accompanying behavioral or psychological disturbance *(no additional medical code)*
F03.90	Major neurocognitive disorder possibly due to vascular disease, Unspecified severity, Without accompanying behavioral or psychological disturbance *(no additional medical code)*
F03.90	Major neurocognitive disorder due to unknown etiology, Unspecified severity, Without accompanying behavioral or psychological disturbance *(no additional medical code)*
F03.911	Major neurocognitive disorder due to possible Alzheimer's disease, Unspecified severity, With agitation *(no additional medical code)*
F03.911	Major neurocognitive disorder due to possible frontotemporal degeneration, Unspecified severity, With agitation *(no additional medical code)*
F03.911	Major neurocognitive disorder with possible Lewy bodies, Unspecified severity, With agitation *(no additional medical code)*
F03.911	Major neurocognitive disorder possibly due to Parkinson's disease, Unspecified severity, With agitation *(no additional medical code)*
F03.911	Major neurocognitive disorder possibly due to vascular disease, Unspecified severity, With agitation *(no additional medical code)*
F03.911	Major neurocognitive disorder due to unknown etiology, Unspecified severity, With agitation *(no additional medical code)*

ICD-10-CM Disorder, condition, or problem

F03.918   Major neurocognitive disorder due to possible
            Alzheimer's disease, Unspecified severity, With
            other behavioral or psychological disturbance
            (no additional medical code)

F03.918   Major neurocognitive disorder due to possible
            frontotemporal degeneration, Unspecified
            severity, With other behavioral or psychological
            disturbance *(no additional medical code)*

F03.918   Major neurocognitive disorder with possible Lewy
            bodies, Unspecified severity, With other
            behavioral or psychological disturbance
            (no additional medical code)

F03.918   Major neurocognitive disorder possibly due to
            Parkinson's disease, Unspecified severity, With
            other behavioral or psychological disturbance
            (no additional medical code)

F03.918   Major neurocognitive disorder possibly due to
            vascular disease, Unspecified severity, With other
            behavioral or psychological disturbance
            (no additional medical code)

F03.918   Major neurocognitive disorder due to unknown
            etiology, Unspecified severity, With other
            behavioral or psychological disturbance
            (no additional medical code)

F03.92   Major neurocognitive disorder due to possible
            Alzheimer's disease, Unspecified severity, With
            psychotic disturbance *(no additional medical code)*

F03.92   Major neurocognitive disorder due to possible
            frontotemporal degeneration, Unspecified
            severity, With psychotic disturbance *(no additional
            medical code)*

ICD-10-CM	Disorder, condition, or problem
F03.92	Major neurocognitive disorder with possible Lewy bodies, Unspecified severity, With psychotic disturbance *(no additional medical code)*
F03.92	Major neurocognitive disorder possibly due to Parkinson's disease, Unspecified severity, With psychotic disturbance *(no additional medical code)*
F03.92	Major neurocognitive disorder possibly due to vascular disease, Unspecified severity, With psychotic disturbance *(no additional medical code)*
F03.92	Major neurocognitive disorder due to unknown etiology, Unspecified severity, With psychotic disturbance *(no additional medical code)*
F03.93	Major neurocognitive disorder due to possible Alzheimer's disease, Unspecified severity, With mood symptoms *(no additional medical code)*
F03.93	Major neurocognitive disorder due to possible frontotemporal degeneration, Unspecified severity, With mood symptoms *(no additional medical code)*
F03.93	Major neurocognitive disorder with possible Lewy bodies, Unspecified severity, With mood symptoms *(no additional medical code)*
F03.93	Major neurocognitive disorder possibly due to Parkinson's disease, Unspecified severity, With mood symptoms *(no additional medical code)*
F03.93	Major neurocognitive disorder possibly due to vascular disease, Unspecified severity, With mood symptoms *(no additional medical code)*
F03.93	Major neurocognitive disorder due to unknown etiology, Unspecified severity, With mood symptoms *(no additional medical code)*

ICD-10-CM	Disorder, condition, or problem
F03.94	Major neurocognitive disorder due to possible Alzheimer's disease, Unspecified severity, With anxiety *(no additional medical code)*
F03.94	Major neurocognitive disorder due to possible frontotemporal degeneration, Unspecified severity, With anxiety *(no additional medical code)*
F03.94	Major neurocognitive disorder with possible Lewy bodies, Unspecified severity, With anxiety *(no additional medical code)*
F03.94	Major neurocognitive disorder possibly due to Parkinson's disease, Unspecified severity, With anxiety *(no additional medical code)*
F03.94	Major neurocognitive disorder possibly due to vascular disease, Unspecified severity, With anxiety *(no additional medical code)*
F03.94	Major neurocognitive disorder due to unknown etiology, Unspecified severity, With anxiety *(no additional medical code)*
F03.A0	Major neurocognitive disorder due to possible Alzheimer's disease, Mild, Without accompanying behavioral or psychological disturbance *(no additional medical code)*
F03.A0	Major neurocognitive disorder due to possible frontotemporal degeneration, Mild, Without accompanying behavioral or psychological disturbance *(no additional medical code)*
F03.A0	Major neurocognitive disorder with possible Lewy bodies, Mild, Without accompanying behavioral or psychological disturbance *(no additional medical code)*
F03.A0	Major neurocognitive disorder possibly due to Parkinson's disease, Mild, Without accompanying behavioral or psychological disturbance *(no additional medical code)*

ICD-10-CM   Disorder, condition, or problem

F03.A0	Major neurocognitive disorder possibly due to vascular disease, Mild, Without accompanying behavioral or psychological disturbance *(no additional medical code)*
F03.A0	Major neurocognitive disorder due to unknown etiology, Mild, Without accompanying behavioral or psychological disturbance *(no additional medical code)*
F03.A11	Major neurocognitive disorder due to possible Alzheimer's disease, Mild, With agitation *(no additional medical code)*
F03.A11	Major neurocognitive disorder due to possible frontotemporal degeneration, Mild, With agitation *(no additional medical code)*
F03.A11	Major neurocognitive disorder with possible Lewy bodies, Mild, With agitation *(no additional medical code)*
F03.A11	Major neurocognitive disorder possibly due to Parkinson's disease, Mild, With agitation *(no additional medical code)*
F03.A11	Major neurocognitive disorder possibly due to vascular disease, Mild, With agitation *(no additional medical code)*
F03.A11	Major neurocognitive disorder due to unknown etiology, Mild, With agitation *(no additional medical code)*
F03.A18	Major neurocognitive disorder due to possible Alzheimer's disease, Mild, With other behavioral or psychological disturbance *(no additional medical code)*
F03.A18	Major neurocognitive disorder due to possible frontotemporal degeneration, Mild, With other behavioral or psychological disturbance *(no additional medical code)*

ICD-10-CM	Disorder, condition, or problem
F03.A18	Major neurocognitive disorder with possible Lewy bodies, Mild, With other behavioral or psychological disturbance *(no additional medical code)*
F03.A18	Major neurocognitive disorder possibly due to Parkinson's disease, Mild, With other behavioral or psychological disturbance *(no additional medical code)*
F03.A18	Major neurocognitive disorder possibly due to vascular disease, Mild, With other behavioral or psychological disturbance *(no additional medical code)*
F03.A18	Major neurocognitive disorder due to unknown etiology, Mild, With other behavioral or psychological disturbance *(no additional medical code)*
F03.A2	Major neurocognitive disorder due to possible Alzheimer's disease, Mild, With psychotic disturbance *(no additional medical code)*
F03.A2	Major neurocognitive disorder due to possible frontotemporal degeneration, Mild, With psychotic disturbance *(no additional medical code)*
F03.A2	Major neurocognitive disorder with possible Lewy bodies, Mild, With psychotic disturbance *(no additional medical code)*
F03.A2	Major neurocognitive disorder possibly due to Parkinson's disease, Mild, With psychotic disturbance *(no additional medical code)*
F03.A2	Major neurocognitive disorder possibly due to vascular disease, Mild, With psychotic disturbance *(no additional medical code)*

ICD-10-CM	Disorder, condition, or problem
F03.A2	Major neurocognitive disorder due to unknown etiology, Mild, With psychotic disturbance *(no additional medical code)*
F03.A3	Major neurocognitive disorder due to possible Alzheimer's disease, Mild, With mood symptoms *(no additional medical code)*
F03.A3	Major neurocognitive disorder due to possible frontotemporal degeneration, Mild, With mood symptoms *(no additional medical code)*
F03.A3	Major neurocognitive disorder with possible Lewy bodies, Mild, With mood symptoms *(no additional medical code)*
F03.A3	Major neurocognitive disorder possibly due to Parkinson's disease, Mild, With mood symptoms *(no additional medical code)*
F03.A3	Major neurocognitive disorder possibly due to vascular disease, Mild, With mood symptoms *(no additional medical code)*
F03.A3	Major neurocognitive disorder due to unknown etiology, Mild, With mood symptoms *(no additional medical code)*
F03.A4	Major neurocognitive disorder due to possible Alzheimer's disease, Mild, With anxiety *(no additional medical code)*
F03.A4	Major neurocognitive disorder due to possible frontotemporal degeneration, Mild, With anxiety *(no additional medical code)*
F03.A4	Major neurocognitive disorder with possible Lewy bodies, Mild, With anxiety *(no additional medical code)*
F03.A4	Major neurocognitive disorder possibly due to Parkinson's disease, Mild, With anxiety *(no additional medical code)*

ICD-10-CM	Disorder, condition, or problem
F03.A4	Major neurocognitive disorder possibly due to vascular disease, Mild, With anxiety *(no additional medical code)*
F03.A4	Major neurocognitive disorder due to unknown etiology, Mild, With anxiety *(no additional medical code)*
F03.B0	Major neurocognitive disorder due to possible Alzheimer's disease, Moderate, Without accompanying behavioral or psychological disturbance *(no additional medical code)*
F03.B0	Major neurocognitive disorder due to possible frontotemporal degeneration, Moderate, Without accompanying behavioral or psychological disturbance *(no additional medical code)*
F03.B0	Major neurocognitive disorder with possible Lewy bodies, Moderate, Without accompanying behavioral or psychological disturbance *(no additional medical code)*
F03.B0	Major neurocognitive disorder possibly due to Parkinson's disease, Moderate, Without accompanying behavioral or psychological disturbance *(no additional medical code)*
F03.B0	Major neurocognitive disorder possibly due to vascular disease, Moderate, Without accompanying behavioral or psychological disturbance *(no additional medical code)*
F03.B0	Major neurocognitive disorder due to unknown etiology, Moderate, Without accompanying behavioral or psychological disturbance *(no additional medical code)*
F03.B11	Major neurocognitive disorder due to possible Alzheimer's disease, Moderate, With agitation *(no additional medical code)*

ICD-10-CM	Disorder, condition, or problem

F03.B11   Major neurocognitive disorder due to possible frontotemporal degeneration, Moderate, With agitation *(no additional medical code)*

F03.B11   Major neurocognitive disorder with possible Lewy bodies, Moderate, With agitation *(no additional medical code)*

F03.B11   Major neurocognitive disorder possibly due to Parkinson's disease, Moderate, With agitation *(no additional medical code)*

F03.B11   Major neurocognitive disorder possibly due to vascular disease, Moderate, With agitation *(no additional medical code)*

F03.B11   Major neurocognitive disorder due to unknown etiology, Moderate, With agitation *(no additional medical code)*

F03.B18   Major neurocognitive disorder due to possible Alzheimer's disease, Moderate, With other behavioral or psychological disturbance *(no additional medical code)*

F03.B18   Major neurocognitive disorder due to possible frontotemporal degeneration, Moderate, With other behavioral or psychological disturbance *(no additional medical code)*

F03.B18   Major neurocognitive disorder with possible Lewy bodies, Moderate, With other behavioral or psychological disturbance *(no additional medical code)*

F03.B18   Major neurocognitive disorder possibly due to Parkinson's disease, Moderate, With other behavioral or psychological disturbance *(no additional medical code)*

ICD-10-CM　Disorder, condition, or problem

F03.B18	Major neurocognitive disorder possibly due to vascular disease, Moderate, With other behavioral or psychological disturbance *(no additional medical code)*
F03.B18	Major neurocognitive disorder due to unknown etiology, Moderate, With other behavioral or psychological disturbance *(no additional medical code)*
F03.B2	Major neurocognitive disorder due to possible Alzheimer's disease, Moderate, With psychotic disturbance *(no additional medical code)*
F03.B2	Major neurocognitive disorder due to possible frontotemporal degeneration, Moderate, With psychotic disturbance *(no additional medical code)*
F03.B2	Major neurocognitive disorder with possible Lewy bodies, Moderate, With psychotic disturbance *(no additional medical code)*
F03.B2	Major neurocognitive disorder possibly due to Parkinson's disease, Moderate, With psychotic disturbance *(no additional medical code)*
F03.B2	Major neurocognitive disorder possibly due to vascular disease, Moderate, With psychotic disturbance *(no additional medical code)*
F03.B2	Major neurocognitive disorder due to unknown etiology, Moderate, With psychotic disturbance *(no additional medical code)*
F03.B3	Major neurocognitive disorder due to possible Alzheimer's disease, Moderate, With mood symptoms *(no additional medical code)*
F03.B3	Major neurocognitive disorder due to possible frontotemporal degeneration, Moderate, With mood symptoms *(no additional medical code)*

ICD-10-CM   Disorder, condition, or problem

F03.B3   Major neurocognitive disorder with possible Lewy
           bodies, Moderate, With mood symptoms
           (no additional medical code)

F03.B3   Major neurocognitive disorder possibly due to
           Parkinson's disease, Moderate, With mood
           symptoms *(no additional medical code)*

F03.B3   Major neurocognitive disorder possibly due to
           vascular disease, Moderate, With mood
           symptoms *(no additional medical code)*

F03.B3   Major neurocognitive disorder due to unknown
           etiology, Moderate, With mood symptoms
           (no additional medical code)

F03.B4   Major neurocognitive disorder due to possible
           Alzheimer's disease, Moderate, With anxiety
           (no additional medical code)

F03.B4   Major neurocognitive disorder due to possible
           frontotemporal degeneration, Moderate, With
           anxiety *(no additional medical code)*

F03.B4   Major neurocognitive disorder with possible Lewy
           bodies, Moderate, With anxiety *(no additional
           medical code)*

F03.B4   Major neurocognitive disorder possibly due to
           Parkinson's disease, Moderate, With anxiety
           (no additional medical code)

F03.B4   Major neurocognitive disorder possibly due to
           vascular disease, Moderate, With anxiety
           (no additional medical code)

F03.B4   Major neurocognitive disorder due to unknown
           etiology, Moderate, With anxiety *(no additional
           medical code)*

ICD-10-CM	Disorder, condition, or problem
F03.C0	Major neurocognitive disorder due to possible Alzheimer's disease, Severe, Without accompanying behavioral or psychological disturbance *(no additional medical code)*
F03.C0	Major neurocognitive disorder due to possible frontotemporal degeneration, Severe, Without accompanying behavioral or psychological disturbance *(no additional medical code)*
F03.C0	Major neurocognitive disorder with possible Lewy bodies, Severe, Without accompanying behavioral or psychological disturbance *(no additional medical code)*
F03.C0	Major neurocognitive disorder possibly due to Parkinson's disease, Severe, Without accompanying behavioral or psychological disturbance *(no additional medical code)*
F03.C0	Major neurocognitive disorder possibly due to vascular disease, Severe, Without accompanying behavioral or psychological disturbance *(no additional medical code)*
F03.C0	Major neurocognitive disorder due to unknown etiology, Severe, Without accompanying behavioral or psychological disturbance *(no additional medical code)*
F03.C11	Major neurocognitive disorder due to possible Alzheimer's disease, Severe, With agitation *(no additional medical code)*
F03.C11	Major neurocognitive disorder due to possible frontotemporal degeneration, Severe, With agitation *(no additional medical code)*
F03.C11	Major neurocognitive disorder with possible Lewy bodies, Severe, With agitation *(no additional medical code)*

ICD-10-CM	Disorder, condition, or problem
F03.C11	Major neurocognitive disorder possibly due to Parkinson's disease, Severe, With agitation *(no additional medical code)*
F03.C11	Major neurocognitive disorder possibly due to vascular disease, Severe, With agitation *(no additional medical code)*
F03.C11	Major neurocognitive disorder due to unknown etiology, Severe, With agitation *(no additional medical code)*
F03.C18	Major neurocognitive disorder due to possible Alzheimer's disease, Severe, With other behavioral or psychological disturbance *(no additional medical code)*
F03.C18	Major neurocognitive disorder due to possible frontotemporal degeneration, Severe, With other behavioral or psychological disturbance *(no additional medical code)*
F03.C18	Major neurocognitive disorder with possible Lewy bodies, Severe, With other behavioral or psychological disturbance *(no additional medical code)*
F03.C18	Major neurocognitive disorder possibly due to Parkinson's disease, Severe, With other behavioral or psychological disturbance *(no additional medical code)*
F03.C18	Major neurocognitive disorder possibly due to vascular disease, Severe, With other behavioral or psychological disturbance *(no additional medical code)*
F03.C18	Major neurocognitive disorder due to unknown etiology, Severe, With other behavioral or psychological disturbance *(no additional medical code)*
F03.C2	Major neurocognitive disorder due to possible Alzheimer's disease, Severe, With psychotic disturbance *(no additional medical code)*

ICD-10-CM	Disorder, condition, or problem
F03.C2	Major neurocognitive disorder due to possible frontotemporal degeneration, Severe, With psychotic disturbance *(no additional medical code)*
F03.C2	Major neurocognitive disorder with possible Lewy bodies, Severe, With psychotic disturbance *(no additional medical code)*
F03.C2	Major neurocognitive disorder possibly due to Parkinson's disease, Severe, With psychotic disturbance *(no additional medical code)*
F03.C2	Major neurocognitive disorder possibly due to vascular disease, Severe, With psychotic disturbance *(no additional medical code))*
F03.C2	Major neurocognitive disorder due to unknown etiology, Severe, With psychotic disturbance *(no additional medical code)*
F03.C3	Major neurocognitive disorder due to possible Alzheimer's disease, Severe, With mood symptoms *(no additional medical code)*
F03.C3	Major neurocognitive disorder due to possible frontotemporal degeneration, Severe, With mood symptoms *(no additional medical code)*
F03.C3	Major neurocognitive disorder with possible Lewy bodies, Severe, With mood symptoms *(no additional medical code)*
F03.C3	Major neurocognitive disorder possibly due to Parkinson's disease, Severe, With mood symptoms *(no additional medical code)*
F03.C3	Major neurocognitive disorder possibly due to vascular disease, Severe, With mood symptoms *(no additional medical code)*
F03.C3	Major neurocognitive disorder due to unknown etiology, Severe, With mood symptoms *(no additional medical code)*

ICD-10-CM	Disorder, condition, or problem
F03.C4	Major neurocognitive disorder due to possible Alzheimer's disease, Severe, With anxiety *(no additional medical code)*
F03.C4	Major neurocognitive disorder due to possible frontotemporal degeneration, Severe, With anxiety *(no additional medical code)*
F03.C4	Major neurocognitive disorder with possible Lewy bodies, Severe, With anxiety *(no additional medical code)*
F03.C4	Major neurocognitive disorder possibly due to Parkinson's disease, Severe, With anxiety *(no additional medical code)*
F03.C4	Major neurocognitive disorder possibly due to vascular disease, Severe, With anxiety *(no additional medical code)*
F03.C4	Major neurocognitive disorder due to unknown etiology, Severe, With anxiety *(no additional medical code)*
F05	Delirium due to another medical condition
F05	Delirium due to multiple etiologies
F05	Other specified delirium
F05	Unspecified delirium
F06.0	Psychotic disorder due to another medical condition, With hallucinations
F06.1	Catatonia associated with another mental disorder (catatonia specifier)
F06.1	Catatonic disorder due to another medical condition
F06.1	Unspecified catatonia (*code first* R29.818 other symptoms involving nervous and musculoskeletal systems)

ICD-10-CM	Disorder, condition, or problem
F06.2	Psychotic disorder due to another medical condition, With delusions
F06.31	Depressive disorder due to another medical condition, With depressive features
F06.32	Depressive disorder due to another medical condition, With major depressive–like episode
F06.33	Bipolar and related disorder due to another medical condition, With manic features
F06.33	Bipolar and related disorder due to another medical condition, With manic- or hypomanic-like episode
F06.34	Bipolar and related disorder due to another medical condition, With mixed features
F06.34	Depressive disorder due to another medical condition, With mixed features
F06.4	Anxiety disorder due to another medical condition
F06.70	Mild neurocognitive disorder due to another medical condition (*code first* the other medical condition), Without behavioral disturbance
F06.70	Mild neurocognitive disorder due to HIV infection (*code first* B20 HIV infection), Without behavioral disturbance
F06.70	Mild neurocognitive disorder due to Huntington's disease (*code first* G10 Huntington's disease), Without behavioral disturbance
F06.70	Mild neurocognitive disorder due to multiple etiologies (*code first* the other medical etiologies), Without behavioral disturbance
F06.70	Mild neurocognitive disorder due to prion disease (*code first* A81.9 prion disease), Without behavioral disturbance

ICD-10-CM Disorder, condition, or problem

ICD-10-CM	Disorder, condition, or problem
F06.70	Mild neurocognitive disorder due to probable Alzheimer's disease (*code first* G30.9 Alzheimer's disease), Without behavioral disturbance
F06.70	Mild neurocognitive disorder due to probable frontotemporal degeneration (*code first* G31.09 frontotemporal degeneration), Without behavioral disturbance
F06.70	Mild neurocognitive disorder with probable Lewy bodies (*code first* G31.83 Lewy body disease), Without behavioral disturbance
F06.70	Mild neurocognitive disorder probably due to Parkinson's disease (*code first* G20.C Parkinson's disease), Without behavioral disturbance
F06.70	Mild neurocognitive disorder probably due to vascular disease (*code first* I67.9 for cerebrovascular disease), Without behavioral disturbance
F06.70	Mild neurocognitive disorder due to traumatic brain injury (*code first* S06.2XAS diffuse traumatic brain injury with loss of consciousness of unspecified duration, sequela), Without behavioral disturbance
F06.71	Mild neurocognitive disorder due to another medical condition (*code first* the other medical condition), With behavioral disturbance
F06.71	Mild neurocognitive disorder due to HIV infection (*code first* B20 HIV infection), With behavioral disturbance
F06.71	Mild neurocognitive disorder due to Huntington's disease (*code first* G10 Huntington's disease), With behavioral disturbance

ICD-10-CM	Disorder, condition, or problem
F06.71	Mild neurocognitive disorder due to multiple etiologies (*code first* the other medical etiologies), With behavioral disturbance
F06.71	Mild neurocognitive disorder due to prion disease (*code first* A81.9 prion disease), With behavioral disturbance
F06.71	Mild neurocognitive disorder due to probable Alzheimer's disease (*code first* G30.9 Alzheimer's disease), With behavioral disturbance
F06.71	Mild neurocognitive disorder due to probable frontotemporal degeneration (*code first* G31.09 frontotemporal degeneration), With behavioral disturbance
F06.71	Mild neurocognitive disorder with probable Lewy bodies (*code first* G31.83 Lewy body disease), With behavioral disturbance
F06.71	Mild neurocognitive disorder probably due to Parkinson's disease (*code first* G20.C Parkinson's disease), With behavioral disturbance
F06.71	Mild neurocognitive disorder probably due to vascular disease (*code first* I67.9 for cerebrovascular disease), With behavioral disturbance
F06.71	Mild neurocognitive disorder due to traumatic brain injury (*code first* S06.2XAS diffuse traumatic brain injury with loss of consciousness of unspecified duration, sequela), With behavioral disturbance
F06.8	Obsessive-compulsive and related disorder due to another medical condition
F06.8	Other specified mental disorder due to another medical condition

ICD-10-CM Disorder, condition, or problem

F07.0	Personality change due to another medical condition
F09	Unspecified mental disorder due to another medical condition
F10.10	Alcohol use disorder, Mild
F10.11	Alcohol use disorder, Mild, In early remission
F10.11	Alcohol use disorder, Mild, In sustained remission
F10.120	Alcohol intoxication, With mild use disorder
F10.121	Alcohol intoxication delirium, With mild use disorder
F10.130	Alcohol withdrawal, Without perceptual disturbances, With mild use disorder
F10.131	Alcohol withdrawal delirium, With mild use disorder
F10.132	Alcohol withdrawal, With perceptual disturbances, With mild use disorder
F10.14	Alcohol-induced bipolar and related disorder, With mild use disorder
F10.14	Alcohol-induced depressive disorder, With mild use disorder
F10.159	Alcohol-induced psychotic disorder, With mild use disorder
F10.180	Alcohol-induced anxiety disorder, With mild use disorder
F10.181	Alcohol-induced sexual dysfunction, With mild use disorder
F10.182	Alcohol-induced sleep disorder, With mild use disorder

ICD-10-CM	Disorder, condition, or problem
F10.188	Alcohol-induced mild neurocognitive disorder, With mild use disorder
F10.20	Alcohol use disorder, Moderate
F10.20	Alcohol use disorder, Severe
F10.21	Alcohol use disorder, Moderate, In early remission
F10.21	Alcohol use disorder, Moderate, In sustained remission
F10.21	Alcohol use disorder, Severe, In early remission
F10.21	Alcohol use disorder, Severe, In sustained remission
F10.220	Alcohol intoxication, With moderate or severe use disorder
F10.221	Alcohol intoxication delirium, With moderate or severe use disorder
F10.230	Alcohol withdrawal, Without perceptual disturbances, With moderate or severe use disorder
F10.231	Alcohol withdrawal delirium, With moderate or severe use disorder
F10.232	Alcohol withdrawal, With perceptual disturbances, With moderate or severe use disorder
F10.24	Alcohol-induced bipolar and related disorder, With moderate or severe use disorder
F10.24	Alcohol-induced depressive disorder, With moderate or severe use disorder
F10.259	Alcohol-induced psychotic disorder, With moderate or severe use disorder
F10.26	Alcohol-induced major neurocognitive disorder, Amnestic-confabulatory type, With moderate or severe use disorder

ICD-10-CM Disorder, condition, or problem

F10.27	Alcohol-induced major neurocognitive disorder, Nonamnestic-confabulatory type, With moderate or severe use disorder
F10.280	Alcohol-induced anxiety disorder, With moderate or severe use disorder
F10.281	Alcohol-induced sexual dysfunction, With moderate or severe use disorder
F10.282	Alcohol-induced sleep disorder, With moderate or severe use disorder
F10.288	Alcohol-induced mild neurocognitive disorder, With moderate or severe use disorder
F10.920	Alcohol intoxication, Without use disorder
F10.921	Alcohol intoxication delirium, Without use disorder
F10.930	Alcohol withdrawal, Without perceptual disturbances, Without use disorder
F10.931	Alcohol withdrawal delirium, without use disorder
F10.932	Alcohol withdrawal, With perceptual disturbances, Without use disorder
F10.94	Alcohol-induced bipolar and related disorder, Without use disorder
F10.94	Alcohol-induced depressive disorder, Without use disorder
F10.959	Alcohol-induced psychotic disorder, Without use disorder
F10.96	Alcohol-induced major neurocognitive disorder, Amnestic-confabulatory type, Without use disorder
F10.97	Alcohol-induced major neurocognitive disorder, Nonamnestic-confabulatory type, Without use disorder

ICD-10-CM	Disorder, condition, or problem
F10.980	Alcohol-induced anxiety disorder, Without use disorder
F10.981	Alcohol-induced sexual dysfunction, Without use disorder
F10.982	Alcohol-induced sleep disorder, Without use disorder
F10.988	Alcohol-induced mild neurocognitive disorder, Without use disorder
F10.99	Unspecified alcohol-related disorder
F11.10	Opioid use disorder, Mild
F11.11	Opioid use disorder, Mild, In early remission
F11.11	Opioid use disorder, Mild, In sustained remission
F11.120	Opioid intoxication, Without perceptual disturbances, With mild use disorder
F11.121	Opioid intoxication delirium, With mild use disorder
F11.122	Opioid intoxication, With perceptual disturbances, With mild use disorder
F11.13	Opioid withdrawal, With mild use disorder
F11.14	Opioid-induced depressive disorder, With mild use disorder
F11.181	Opioid-induced sexual dysfunction, With mild use disorder
F11.182	Opioid-induced sleep disorder, With mild use disorder
F11.188	Opioid-induced anxiety disorder, With mild use disorder
F11.188	Opioid withdrawal delirium, With mild use disorder
F11.20	Opioid use disorder, Moderate

ICD-10-CM Disorder, condition, or problem

ICD-10-CM	Disorder, condition, or problem
F11.20	Opioid use disorder, Severe
F11.21	Opioid use disorder, Moderate, In early remission
F11.21	Opioid use disorder, Moderate, In sustained remission
F11.21	Opioid use disorder, Severe, In early remission
F11.21	Opioid use disorder, Severe, In sustained remission
F11.220	Opioid intoxication, Without perceptual disturbances, With moderate or severe use disorder
F11.221	Opioid intoxication delirium, With moderate or severe use disorder
F11.222	Opioid intoxication, With perceptual disturbances, With moderate or severe use disorder
F11.23	Opioid withdrawal, With moderate or severe use disorder
F11.24	Opioid-induced depressive disorder, With moderate or severe use disorder
F11.281	Opioid-induced sexual dysfunction, With moderate or severe use disorder
F11.282	Opioid-induced sleep disorder, With moderate or severe use disorder
F11.288	Opioid-induced anxiety disorder, With moderate or severe use disorder
F11.288	Opioid withdrawal delirium, With moderate or severe use disorder
F11.920	Opioid intoxication, Without perceptual disturbances, Without use disorder
F11.921	Opioid-induced delirium (opioid medication taken as prescribed)
F11.921	Opioid intoxication delirium, Without use disorder

ICD-10-CM	Disorder, condition, or problem
F11.922	Opioid intoxication, With perceptual disturbances, Without use disorder
F11.93	Opioid withdrawal, Without use disorder
F11.94	Opioid-induced depressive disorder, Without use disorder
F11.981	Opioid-induced sexual dysfunction, Without use disorder
F11.982	Opioid-induced sleep disorder, Without use disorder
F11.988	Opioid-induced anxiety disorder, Without use disorder
F11.988	Opioid-induced delirium (during withdrawal from opioid medication taken as prescribed)
F11.988	Opioid withdrawal delirium, Without use disorder
F11.99	Unspecified opioid-related disorder
F12.10	Cannabis use disorder, Mild
F12.11	Cannabis use disorder, Mild, In early remission
F12.11	Cannabis use disorder, Mild, In sustained remission
F12.120	Cannabis intoxication, Without perceptual disturbances, With mild use disorder
F12.121	Cannabis intoxication delirium, With mild use disorder
F12.122	Cannabis intoxication, With perceptual disturbances, With mild use disorder
F12.13	Cannabis withdrawal, With mild use disorder
F12.159	Cannabis-induced psychotic disorder, With mild use disorder
F12.180	Cannabis-induced anxiety disorder, With mild use disorder

ICD-10-CM   Disorder, condition, or problem

F12.188	Cannabis-induced sleep disorder, With mild use disorder
F12.20	Cannabis use disorder, Moderate
F12.20	Cannabis use disorder, Severe
F12.21	Cannabis use disorder, Moderate, In early remission
F12.21	Cannabis use disorder, Moderate, In sustained remission
F12.21	Cannabis use disorder, Severe, In early remission
F12.21	Cannabis use disorder, Severe, In sustained remission
F12.220	Cannabis intoxication, Without perceptual disturbances, With moderate or severe use disorder
F12.221	Cannabis intoxication delirium, With moderate or severe use disorder
F12.222	Cannabis intoxication, With perceptual disturbances, With moderate or severe use disorder
F12.23	Cannabis withdrawal, With moderate or severe use disorder
F12.259	Cannabis-induced psychotic disorder, With moderate or severe use disorder
F12.280	Cannabis-induced anxiety disorder, With moderate or severe use disorder
F12.288	Cannabis-induced sleep disorder, With moderate or severe use disorder
F12.920	Cannabis intoxication, Without perceptual disturbances, Without use disorder
F12.921	Cannabis intoxication delirium, Without use disorder

ICD-10-CM	Disorder, condition, or problem
F12.921	Pharmaceutical cannabis receptor agonist–induced delirium (pharmaceutical cannabis receptor agonist medication taken as prescribed)
F12.922	Cannabis intoxication, With perceptual disturbances, Without use disorder
F12.93	Cannabis withdrawal, Without use disorder
F12.959	Cannabis-induced psychotic disorder, Without use disorder
F12.980	Cannabis-induced anxiety disorder, Without use disorder
F12.988	Cannabis-induced sleep disorder, Without use disorder
F12.99	Unspecified cannabis-related disorder
F13.10	Sedative, hypnotic, or anxiolytic use disorder, Mild
F13.11	Sedative, hypnotic, or anxiolytic use disorder, Mild, In early remission
F13.11	Sedative, hypnotic, or anxiolytic use disorder, Mild, In sustained remission
F13.120	Sedative, hypnotic, or anxiolytic intoxication, With mild use disorder
F13.121	Sedative, hypnotic, or anxiolytic intoxication delirium, With mild use disorder
F13.130	Sedative, hypnotic, or anxiolytic withdrawal, Without perceptual disturbances, With mild use disorder
F13.131	Sedative, hypnotic, or anxiolytic withdrawal delirium, With mild use disorder
F13.132	Sedative, hypnotic, or anxiolytic withdrawal, With perceptual disturbances, With mild use disorder
F13.14	Sedative-, hypnotic-, or anxiolytic-induced bipolar and related disorder, With mild use disorder

ICD-10-CM Disorder, condition, or problem

F13.14	Sedative-, hypnotic-, or anxiolytic-induced depressive disorder, With mild use disorder
F13.159	Sedative-, hypnotic-, or anxiolytic-induced psychotic disorder, With mild use disorder
F13.180	Sedative-, hypnotic-, or anxiolytic-induced anxiety disorder, With mild use disorder
F13.181	Sedative-, hypnotic-, or anxiolytic-induced sexual dysfunction, With mild use disorder
F13.182	Sedative-, hypnotic-, or anxiolytic-induced sleep disorder, With mild use disorder
F13.188	Sedative-, hypnotic-, or anxiolytic-induced mild neurocognitive disorder, With mild use disorder
F13.20	Sedative, hypnotic, or anxiolytic use disorder, Moderate
F13.20	Sedative, hypnotic, or anxiolytic use disorder, Severe
F13.21	Sedative, hypnotic, or anxiolytic use disorder, Moderate, In early remission
F13.21	Sedative, hypnotic, or anxiolytic use disorder, Moderate, In sustained remission
F13.21	Sedative, hypnotic, or anxiolytic use disorder, Severe, In early remission
F13.21	Sedative, hypnotic, or anxiolytic use disorder, Severe, In sustained remission
F13.220	Sedative, hypnotic, or anxiolytic intoxication, With moderate or severe use disorder
F13.221	Sedative, hypnotic, or anxiolytic intoxication delirium, With moderate or severe use disorder
F13.230	Sedative, hypnotic, or anxiolytic withdrawal, Without perceptual disturbances, With moderate or severe use disorder

ICD-10-CM	Disorder, condition, or problem
F13.231	Sedative, hypnotic, or anxiolytic withdrawal delirium, With moderate or severe use disorder
F13.232	Sedative, hypnotic, or anxiolytic withdrawal, With perceptual disturbances, With moderate or severe use disorder
F13.24	Sedative-, hypnotic-, or anxiolytic-induced bipolar and related disorder, With moderate or severe use disorder
F13.24	Sedative-, hypnotic-, or anxiolytic-induced depressive disorder, With moderate or severe use disorder
F13.259	Sedative-, hypnotic-, or anxiolytic-induced psychotic disorder, With moderate or severe use disorder
F13.27	Sedative-, hypnotic-, or anxiolytic-induced major neurocognitive disorder, With moderate or severe use disorder
F13.280	Sedative-, hypnotic-, or anxiolytic-induced anxiety disorder, With moderate or severe use disorder
F13.281	Sedative-, hypnotic-, or anxiolytic-induced sexual dysfunction, With moderate or severe use disorder
F13.282	Sedative-, hypnotic-, or anxiolytic-induced sleep disorder, With moderate or severe use disorder
F13.288	Sedative-, hypnotic-, or anxiolytic-induced mild neurocognitive disorder, With moderate or severe use disorder
F13.920	Sedative, hypnotic, or anxiolytic intoxication, Without use disorder
F13.921	Sedative-, hypnotic-, or anxiolytic-induced delirium (sedative, hypnotic, or anxiolytic medication taken as prescribed)

ICD-10-CM	Disorder, condition, or problem
F13.921	Sedative, hypnotic, or anxiolytic intoxication delirium, Without use disorder
F13.930	Sedative, hypnotic, or anxiolytic withdrawal, Without perceptual disturbances, Without use disorder
F13.931	Sedative, hypnotic, or anxiolytic–induced delirium (during withdrawal from sedative, hypnotic, or anxiolytic medication taken as prescribed)
F13.931	Sedative, hypnotic, or anxiolytic withdrawal delirium, Without use disorder
F13.932	Sedative, hypnotic, or anxiolytic withdrawal, With perceptual disturbances, Without use disorder
F13.94	Sedative-, hypnotic-, or anxiolytic-induced bipolar and related disorder, Without use disorder
F13.94	Sedative-, hypnotic-, or anxiolytic-induced depressive disorder, Without use disorder
F13.959	Sedative-, hypnotic-, or anxiolytic-induced psychotic disorder, Without use disorder
F13.97	Sedative-, hypnotic-, or anxiolytic-induced major neurocognitive disorder, Without use disorder
F13.980	Sedative-, hypnotic-, or anxiolytic-induced anxiety disorder, Without use disorder
F13.981	Sedative-, hypnotic-, or anxiolytic-induced sexual dysfunction, Without use disorder
F13.982	Sedative-, hypnotic-, or anxiolytic-induced sleep disorder, Without use disorder
F13.988	Sedative-, hypnotic-, or anxiolytic-induced mild neurocognitive disorder, Without use disorder
F13.99	Unspecified sedative-, hypnotic-, or anxiolytic-related disorder
F14.10	Cocaine use disorder, Mild

ICD-10-CM	Disorder, condition, or problem
F14.11	Cocaine use disorder, Mild, In early remission
F14.11	Cocaine use disorder, Mild, In sustained remission
F14.120	Cocaine intoxication, Without perceptual disturbances, With mild use disorder
F14.121	Cocaine intoxication delirium, With mild use disorder
F14.122	Cocaine intoxication, With perceptual disturbances, With mild use disorder
F14.13	Cocaine withdrawal, With mild use disorder
F14.14	Cocaine-induced bipolar and related disorder, With mild use disorder
F14.14	Cocaine-induced depressive disorder, With mild use disorder
F14.159	Cocaine-induced psychotic disorder, With mild use disorder
F14.180	Cocaine-induced anxiety disorder, With mild use disorder
F14.181	Cocaine-induced sexual dysfunction, With mild use disorder
F14.182	Cocaine-induced sleep disorder, With mild use disorder
F14.188	Cocaine-induced mild neurocognitive disorder, With mild use disorder
F14.188	Cocaine-induced obsessive-compulsive and related disorder, With mild use disorder
F14.20	Cocaine use disorder, Moderate
F14.20	Cocaine use disorder, Severe
F14.21	Cocaine use disorder, Moderate, In early remission
F14.21	Cocaine use disorder, Moderate, In sustained remission

ICD-10-CM	Disorder, condition, or problem
F14.21	Cocaine use disorder, Severe, In early remission
F14.21	Cocaine use disorder, Severe, In sustained remission
F14.220	Cocaine intoxication, Without perceptual disturbances, With moderate or severe use disorder
F14.221	Cocaine intoxication delirium, With moderate or severe use disorder
F14.222	Cocaine intoxication, With perceptual disturbances, With moderate or severe use disorder
F14.23	Cocaine withdrawal, With moderate or severe use disorder
F14.24	Cocaine-induced bipolar and related disorder, With moderate or severe use disorder
F14.24	Cocaine-induced depressive disorder, With moderate or severe use disorder
F14.259	Cocaine-induced psychotic disorder, With moderate or severe use disorder
F14.280	Cocaine-induced anxiety disorder, With moderate or severe use disorder
F14.281	Cocaine-induced sexual dysfunction, With moderate or severe use disorder
F14.282	Cocaine-induced sleep disorder, With moderate or severe use disorder
F14.288	Cocaine-induced mild neurocognitive disorder, With moderate or severe use disorder
F14.288	Cocaine-induced obsessive-compulsive and related disorder, With moderate or severe use disorder
F14.920	Cocaine intoxication, Without perceptual disturbances, Without use disorder

ICD-10-CM   Disorder, condition, or problem

F14.921	Cocaine intoxication delirium, Without use disorder
F14.922	Cocaine intoxication, With perceptual disturbances, Without use disorder
F14.93	Cocaine withdrawal, Without use disorder
F14.94	Cocaine-induced bipolar and related disorder, Without use disorder
F14.94	Cocaine-induced depressive disorder, Without use disorder
F14.959	Cocaine-induced psychotic disorder, Without use disorder
F14.980	Cocaine-induced anxiety disorder, Without use disorder
F14.981	Cocaine-induced sexual dysfunction, Without use disorder
F14.982	Cocaine-induced sleep disorder, Without use disorder
F14.988	Cocaine-induced mild neurocognitive disorder, Without use disorder
F14.988	Cocaine-induced obsessive-compulsive and related disorder, Without use disorder
F14.99	Unspecified cocaine-related disorder
F15.10	Amphetamine-type substance use disorder, Mild
F15.10	Other or unspecified stimulant use disorder, Mild
F15.11	Amphetamine-type substance use disorder, Mild, In early remission
F15.11	Amphetamine-type substance use disorder, Mild, In sustained remission
F15.11	Other or unspecified stimulant use disorder, Mild, In early remission

ICD-10-CM	Disorder, condition, or problem
F15.11	Other or unspecified stimulant use disorder, Mild, In sustained remission
F15.120	Amphetamine-type substance intoxication, Without perceptual disturbances, With mild use disorder
F15.120	Other stimulant intoxication, Without perceptual disturbances, With mild use disorder
F15.121	Amphetamine-type substance (or other stimulant) intoxication delirium, With mild use disorder
F15.122	Amphetamine-type substance intoxication, With perceptual disturbances, With mild use disorder
F15.122	Other stimulant intoxication, With perceptual disturbances, With mild use disorder
F15.13	Amphetamine-type substance withdrawal, With mild use disorder
F15.13	Other stimulant withdrawal, With mild use disorder
F15.14	Amphetamine-type substance (or other stimulant)–induced bipolar and related disorder, With mild use disorder
F15.14	Amphetamine-type substance (or other stimulant)–induced depressive disorder, With mild use disorder
F15.159	Amphetamine-type substance (or other stimulant)–induced psychotic disorder, With mild use disorder
F15.180	Amphetamine-type substance (or other stimulant)–induced anxiety disorder, With mild use disorder
F15.181	Amphetamine-type substance (or other stimulant)–induced sexual dysfunction, With mild use disorder

ICD-10-CM	Disorder, condition, or problem
F15.182	Amphetamine-type substance (or other stimulant)–induced sleep disorder, With mild use disorder
F15.188	Amphetamine-type substance (or other stimulant)–induced mild neurocognitive disorder, With mild use disorder
F15.188	Amphetamine-type substance (or other stimulant)–induced obsessive-compulsive and related disorder, With mild use disorder
F15.20	Amphetamine-type substance use disorder, Moderate
F15.20	Amphetamine-type substance use disorder, Severe
F15.20	Other or unspecified stimulant use disorder, Moderate
F15.20	Other or unspecified stimulant use disorder, Severe
F15.21	Amphetamine-type substance use disorder, Moderate, In early remission
F15.21	Amphetamine-type substance use disorder, Moderate, In sustained remission
F15.21	Amphetamine-type substance use disorder, Severe, In early remission
F15.21	Amphetamine-type substance use disorder, Severe, In sustained remission
F15.21	Other or unspecified stimulant use disorder, Moderate, In early remission
F15.21	Other or unspecified stimulant use disorder, Moderate, In sustained remission
F15.21	Other or unspecified stimulant use disorder, Severe, In early remission
F15.21	Other or unspecified stimulant use disorder, Severe, In sustained remission

ICD-10-CM Disorder, condition, or problem

F15.220	Amphetamine-type substance intoxication, Without perceptual disturbances, With moderate or severe use disorder
F15.220	Other stimulant intoxication, Without perceptual disturbances, With moderate or severe use disorder
F15.221	Amphetamine-type substance (or other stimulant) intoxication delirium, With moderate or severe use disorder
F15.222	Amphetamine-type substance intoxication, With perceptual disturbances, With moderate or severe use disorder
F15.222	Other stimulant intoxication, With perceptual disturbances, With moderate or severe use disorder
F15.23	Amphetamine-type substance withdrawal, With moderate or severe use disorder
F15.23	Other stimulant withdrawal, With moderate or severe use disorder
F15.24	Amphetamine-type substance (or other stimulant)–induced bipolar and related disorder, With moderate or severe use disorder
F15.24	Amphetamine-type substance (or other stimulant)–induced depressive disorder, With moderate or severe use disorder
F15.259	Amphetamine-type substance (or other stimulant)–induced psychotic disorder, With moderate or severe use disorder
F15.280	Amphetamine-type substance (or other stimulant)–induced anxiety disorder, With moderate or severe use disorder

ICD-10-CM	Disorder, condition, or problem
F15.281	Amphetamine-type substance (or other stimulant)–induced sexual dysfunction, With moderate or severe use disorder
F15.282	Amphetamine-type substance (or other stimulant)–induced sleep disorder, With moderate or severe use disorder
F15.288	Amphetamine-type substance (or other stimulant)–induced mild neurocognitive disorder, With moderate or severe use disorder
F15.288	Amphetamine-type substance (or other stimulant)–induced obsessive-compulsive and related disorder, With moderate or severe use disorder
F15.920	Amphetamine-type substance intoxication, Without perceptual disturbances, Without use disorder
F15.920	Caffeine intoxication
F15.920	Other stimulant intoxication, Without perceptual disturbances, Without use disorder
F15.921	Amphetamine-type (or other stimulant) medication–induced delirium (amphetamine-type or other stimulant medication taken as prescribed)
F15.921	Amphetamine-type substance (or other stimulant) intoxication delirium, Without use disorder
F15.922	Amphetamine-type substance intoxication, With perceptual disturbances, Without use disorder
F15.922	Other stimulant intoxication, With perceptual disturbances, Without use disorder
F15.93	Amphetamine-type substance withdrawal, Without use disorder
F15.93	Caffeine withdrawal
F15.93	Other stimulant withdrawal, Without use disorder

ICD-10-CM Disorder, condition, or problem

F15.94	Amphetamine-type substance (or other stimulant)–induced bipolar and related disorder, Without use disorder
F15.94	Amphetamine-type substance (or other stimulant)–induced depressive disorder, Without use disorder
F15.959	Amphetamine-type substance (or other stimulant)–induced psychotic disorder, Without use disorder
F15.980	Amphetamine-type substance (or other stimulant)–induced anxiety disorder, Without use disorder
F15.980	Caffeine-induced anxiety disorder, Without use disorder
F15.981	Amphetamine-type substance (or other stimulant)–induced sexual dysfunction, Without use disorder
F15.982	Amphetamine-type substance (or other stimulant)–induced sleep disorder, Without use disorder
F15.982	Caffeine-induced sleep disorder, Without use disorder
F15.988	Amphetamine-type substance (or other stimulant)–induced mild neurocognitive disorder, Without use disorder
F15.988	Amphetamine-type substance (or other stimulant)–induced obsessive-compulsive and related disorder, Without use disorder
F15.99	Unspecified amphetamine-type substance-related disorder
F15.99	Unspecified caffeine-related disorder
F15.99	Unspecified other stimulant–related disorder
F16.10	Other hallucinogen use disorder, Mild
F16.10	Phencyclidine use disorder, Mild

ICD-10-CM	Disorder, condition, or problem
F16.11	Other hallucinogen use disorder, Mild, In early remission
F16.11	Other hallucinogen use disorder, Mild, In sustained remission
F16.11	Phencyclidine use disorder, Mild, In early remission
F16.11	Phencyclidine use disorder, Mild, In sustained remission
F16.120	Other hallucinogen intoxication, With mild use disorder
F16.120	Phencyclidine intoxication, With mild use disorder
F16.121	Other hallucinogen intoxication delirium, With mild use disorder
F16.121	Phencyclidine intoxication delirium, With mild use disorder
F16.14	Other hallucinogen–induced bipolar and related disorder, With mild use disorder
F16.14	Other hallucinogen–induced depressive disorder, With mild use disorder
F16.14	Phencyclidine-induced bipolar and related disorder, With mild use disorder
F16.14	Phencyclidine-induced depressive disorder, With mild use disorder
F16.159	Other hallucinogen–induced psychotic disorder, With mild use disorder
F16.159	Phencyclidine-induced psychotic disorder, With mild use disorder
F16.180	Other hallucinogen–induced anxiety disorder, With mild use disorder
F16.180	Phencyclidine-induced anxiety disorder, With mild use disorder

ICD-10-CM Disorder, condition, or problem

ICD-10-CM	Disorder, condition, or problem
F16.20	Other hallucinogen use disorder, Moderate
F16.20	Other hallucinogen use disorder, Severe
F16.20	Phencyclidine use disorder, Moderate
F16.20	Phencyclidine use disorder, Severe
F16.21	Other hallucinogen use disorder, Moderate, In early remission
F16.21	Other hallucinogen use disorder, Moderate, In sustained remission
F16.21	Other hallucinogen use disorder, Severe, In early remission
F16.21	Other hallucinogen use disorder, Severe, In sustained remission
F16.21	Phencyclidine use disorder, Moderate, In early remission
F16.21	Phencyclidine use disorder, Moderate, In sustained remission
F16.21	Phencyclidine use disorder, Severe, In early remission
F16.21	Phencyclidine use disorder, Severe, In sustained remission
F16.220	Other hallucinogen intoxication, With moderate or severe use disorder
F16.220	Phencyclidine intoxication, With moderate or severe use disorder
F16.221	Other hallucinogen intoxication delirium, With moderate or severe use disorder
F16.221	Phencyclidine intoxication delirium, With moderate or severe use disorder
F16.24	Other hallucinogen–induced bipolar and related disorder, With moderate or severe use disorder

ICD-10-CM   Disorder, condition, or problem

ICD-10-CM	Disorder, condition, or problem
F16.24	Other hallucinogen–induced depressive disorder, With moderate or severe use disorder
F16.24	Phencyclidine-induced bipolar and related disorder, With moderate or severe use disorder
F16.24	Phencyclidine-induced depressive disorder, With moderate or severe use disorder
F16.259	Other hallucinogen–induced psychotic disorder, With moderate or severe use disorder
F16.259	Phencyclidine-induced psychotic disorder, With moderate or severe use disorder
F16.280	Other hallucinogen–induced anxiety disorder, With moderate or severe use disorder
F16.280	Phencyclidine-induced anxiety disorder, With moderate or severe use disorder
F16.920	Other hallucinogen intoxication, Without use disorder
F16.920	Phencyclidine intoxication, Without use disorder
F16.921	Ketamine or other hallucinogen–induced delirium (ketamine or other hallucinogen medication taken as prescribed or for medical reasons)
F16.921	Other hallucinogen intoxication delirium, Without use disorder
F16.921	Phencyclidine intoxication delirium, Without use disorder
F16.94	Other hallucinogen–induced bipolar and related disorder, Without use disorder
F16.94	Other hallucinogen–induced depressive disorder, Without use disorder
F16.94	Phencyclidine-induced bipolar and related disorder, Without use disorder

ICD-10-CM   Disorder, condition, or problem

F16.94	Phencyclidine-induced depressive disorder, Without use disorder
F16.959	Other hallucinogen–induced psychotic disorder, Without use disorder
F16.959	Phencyclidine-induced psychotic disorder, Without use disorder
F16.980	Other hallucinogen–induced anxiety disorder, Without use disorder
F16.980	Phencyclidine-induced anxiety disorder, Without use disorder
F16.983	Hallucinogen persisting perception disorder
F16.99	Unspecified hallucinogen-related disorder
F16.99	Unspecified phencyclidine-related disorder
F17.200	Tobacco use disorder, Moderate
F17.200	Tobacco use disorder, Severe
F17.201	Tobacco use disorder, Moderate, In early remission
F17.201	Tobacco use disorder, Moderate, In sustained remission
F17.201	Tobacco use disorder, Severe, In early remission
F17.201	Tobacco use disorder, Severe, In sustained remission
F17.203	Tobacco withdrawal
F17.208	Tobacco-induced sleep disorder, With moderate or severe use disorder
F17.209	Unspecified tobacco-related disorder
F18.10	Inhalant use disorder, Mild
F18.11	Inhalant use disorder, Mild, In early remission
F18.11	Inhalant use disorder, Mild, In sustained remission
F18.120	Inhalant intoxication, With mild use disorder

ICD-10-CM	Disorder, condition, or problem
F18.121	Inhalant intoxication delirium, With mild use disorder
F18.14	Inhalant-induced depressive disorder, With mild use disorder
F18.159	Inhalant-induced psychotic disorder, With mild use disorder
F18.17	Inhalant-induced major neurocognitive disorder, With mild use disorder
F18.180	Inhalant-induced anxiety disorder, With mild use disorder
F18.188	Inhalant-induced mild neurocognitive disorder, With mild use disorder
F18.20	Inhalant use disorder, Moderate
F18.20	Inhalant use disorder, Severe
F18.21	Inhalant use disorder, Moderate, In early remission
F18.21	Inhalant use disorder, Moderate, In sustained remission
F18.21	Inhalant use disorder, Severe, In early remission
F18.21	Inhalant use disorder, Severe, In sustained remission
F18.220	Inhalant intoxication, With moderate or severe use disorder
F18.221	Inhalant intoxication delirium, With moderate or severe use disorder
F18.24	Inhalant-induced depressive disorder, With moderate or severe use disorder
F18.259	Inhalant-induced psychotic disorder, With moderate or severe use disorder
F18.27	Inhalant-induced major neurocognitive disorder, With moderate or severe use disorder

ICD-10-CM Disorder, condition, or problem

ICD-10-CM	Disorder, condition, or problem
F18.280	Inhalant-induced anxiety disorder, With moderate or severe use disorder
F18.288	Inhalant-induced mild neurocognitive disorder, With moderate or severe use disorder
F18.920	Inhalant intoxication, Without use disorder
F18.921	Inhalant intoxication delirium, Without use disorder
F18.94	Inhalant-induced depressive disorder, Without use disorder
F18.959	Inhalant-induced psychotic disorder, Without use disorder
F18.97	Inhalant-induced major neurocognitive disorder, Without use disorder
F18.980	Inhalant-induced anxiety disorder, Without use disorder
F18.988	Inhalant-induced mild neurocognitive disorder, Without use disorder
F18.99	Unspecified inhalant-related disorder
F19.10	Other (or unknown) substance use disorder, Mild
F19.11	Other (or unknown) substance use disorder, Mild, In early remission
F19.11	Other (or unknown) substance use disorder, Mild, In sustained remission
F19.120	Other (or unknown) substance intoxication, Without perceptual disturbances, With mild use disorder
F19.121	Other (or unknown) substance intoxication delirium, With mild use disorder
F19.122	Other (or unknown) substance intoxication, With perceptual disturbances, With mild use disorder

ICD-10-CM	Disorder, condition, or problem
F19.130	Other (or unknown) substance withdrawal, Without perceptual disturbances, With mild use disorder
F19.131	Other (or unknown) substance withdrawal delirium, With mild use disorder
F19.132	Other (or unknown) substance withdrawal, With perceptual disturbances, With mild use disorder
F19.14	Other (or unknown) substance–induced bipolar and related disorder, With mild use disorder
F19.14	Other (or unknown) substance–induced depressive disorder, With mild use disorder
F19.159	Other (or unknown) substance–induced psychotic disorder, With mild use disorder
F19.17	Other (or unknown) substance–induced major neurocognitive disorder, With mild use disorder
F19.180	Other (or unknown) substance–induced anxiety disorder, With mild use disorder
F19.181	Other (or unknown) substance–induced sexual dysfunction, With mild use disorder
F19.182	Other (or unknown) substance–induced sleep disorder, With mild use disorder
F19.188	Other (or unknown) substance–induced mild neurocognitive disorder, With mild use disorder
F19.188	Other (or unknown) substance–induced obsessive-compulsive and related disorder, With mild use disorder
F19.20	Other (or unknown) substance use disorder, Moderate
F19.20	Other (or unknown) substance use disorder, Severe
F19.21	Other (or unknown) substance use disorder, Moderate, In early remission

ICD-10-CM Disorder, condition, or problem

ICD-10-CM	Disorder, condition, or problem
F19.21	Other (or unknown) substance use disorder, Moderate, In sustained remission
F19.21	Other (or unknown) substance use disorder, Severe, In early remission
F19.21	Other (or unknown) substance use disorder, Severe, In sustained remission
F19.220	Other (or unknown) substance intoxication, Without perceptual disturbances, With moderate or severe use disorder
F19.221	Other (or unknown) substance intoxication delirium, With moderate or severe use disorder
F19.222	Other (or unknown) substance intoxication, With perceptual disturbances, With moderate or severe use disorder
F19.230	Other (or unknown) substance withdrawal, Without perceptual disturbances, With moderate or severe use disorder
F19.231	Other (or unknown) substance withdrawal delirium, With moderate or severe use disorder
F19.232	Other (or unknown) substance withdrawal, With perceptual disturbances, With moderate or severe use disorder
F19.24	Other (or unknown) substance–induced bipolar and related disorder, With moderate or severe use disorder
F19.24	Other (or unknown) substance–induced depressive disorder, With moderate or severe use disorder
F19.259	Other (or unknown) substance–induced psychotic disorder, With moderate or severe use disorder
F19.27	Other (or unknown) substance–induced major neurocognitive disorder, With moderate or severe use disorder

ICD-10-CM   Disorder, condition, or problem

F19.280	Other (or unknown) substance–induced anxiety disorder, With moderate or severe use disorder
F19.281	Other (or unknown) substance–induced sexual dysfunction, With moderate or severe use disorder
F19.282	Other (or unknown) substance–induced sleep disorder, With moderate or severe use disorder
F19.288	Other (or unknown) substance–induced mild neurocognitive disorder, With moderate or severe use disorder
F19.288	Other (or unknown) substance–induced obsessive-compulsive and related disorder, With moderate or severe use disorder
F19.920	Other (or unknown) substance intoxication, Without perceptual disturbances, Without use disorder
F19.921	Other (or unknown) medication–induced delirium (other [or unknown] medication taken as prescribed)
F19.921	Other (or unknown) substance intoxication delirium, Without use disorder
F19.922	Other (or unknown) substance intoxication, With perceptual disturbances, Without use disorder
F19.930	Other (or unknown) substance withdrawal, Without perceptual disturbances, Without use disorder
F19.931	Other (or unknown) medication–induced delirium (during withdrawal from other [or unknown] medication taken as prescribed)
F19.931	Other (or unknown) substance withdrawal delirium, Without use disorder

ICD-10-CM	Disorder, condition, or problem
F19.932	Other (or unknown) substance withdrawal, With perceptual disturbances, Without use disorder
F19.94	Other (or unknown) substance–induced bipolar and related disorder, Without use disorder
F19.94	Other (or unknown) substance–induced depressive disorder, Without use disorder
F19.959	Other (or unknown) substance–induced psychotic disorder, Without use disorder
F19.97	Other (or unknown) substance–induced major neurocognitive disorder, Without use disorder
F19.980	Other (or unknown) substance–induced anxiety disorder, Without use disorder
F19.981	Other (or unknown) substance–induced sexual dysfunction, Without use disorder
F19.982	Other (or unknown) substance–induced sleep disorder, Without use disorder
F19.988	Other (or unknown) substance–induced mild neurocognitive disorder, Without use disorder
F19.988	Other (or unknown) substance–induced obsessive-compulsive and related disorder, Without use disorder
F19.99	Unspecified other (or unknown) substance–related disorder
F20.81	Schizophreniform disorder
F20.9	Schizophrenia
F21	Schizotypal personality disorder
F22	Delusional disorder
F23	Brief psychotic disorder
F25.0	Schizoaffective disorder, Bipolar type
F25.1	Schizoaffective disorder, Depressive type

ICD-10-CM	Disorder, condition, or problem
F28	Other specified schizophrenia spectrum and other psychotic disorder
F29	Unspecified schizophrenia spectrum and other psychotic disorder
F31.0	Bipolar I disorder, Current or most recent episode hypomanic
F31.11	Bipolar I disorder, Current or most recent episode manic, Mild
F31.12	Bipolar I disorder, Current or most recent episode manic, Moderate
F31.13	Bipolar I disorder, Current or most recent episode manic, Severe
F31.2	Bipolar I disorder, Current or most recent episode manic, With psychotic features
F31.31	Bipolar I disorder, Current or most recent episode depressed, Mild
F31.32	Bipolar I disorder, Current or most recent episode depressed, Moderate
F31.4	Bipolar I disorder, Current or most recent episode depressed, Severe
F31.5	Bipolar I disorder, Current or most recent episode depressed, With psychotic features
F31.71	Bipolar I disorder, Current or most recent episode hypomanic, In partial remission
F31.72	Bipolar I disorder, Current or most recent episode hypomanic, In full remission
F31.73	Bipolar I disorder, Current or most recent episode manic, In partial remission
F31.74	Bipolar I disorder, Current or most recent episode manic, In full remission

ICD-10-CM Disorder, condition, or problem

F31.75	Bipolar I disorder, Current or most recent episode depressed, In partial remission
F31.76	Bipolar I disorder, Current or most recent episode depressed, In full remission
F31.81	Bipolar II disorder
F31.89	Other specified bipolar and related disorder
F31.9	Bipolar I disorder, Current or most recent episode depressed, Unspecified
F31.9	Bipolar I disorder, Current or most recent episode hypomanic, Unspecified
F31.9	Bipolar I disorder, Current or most recent episode manic, Unspecified
F31.9	Bipolar I disorder, Current or most recent episode unspecified
F31.9	Unspecified bipolar and related disorder
F32.0	Major depressive disorder, Single episode, Mild
F32.1	Major depressive disorder, Single episode, Moderate
F32.2	Major depressive disorder, Single episode, Severe
F32.3	Major depressive disorder, Single episode, With psychotic features
F32.4	Major depressive disorder, Single episode, In partial remission
F32.5	Major depressive disorder, Single episode, In full remission
F32.81	Premenstrual dysphoric disorder
F32.89	Other specified depressive disorder
F32.9	Major depressive disorder, Single episode, Unspecified
F32.A	Unspecified depressive disorder

ICD-10-CM	Disorder, condition, or problem
F33.0	Major depressive disorder, Recurrent episode, Mild
F33.1	Major depressive disorder, Recurrent episode, Moderate
F33.2	Major depressive disorder, Recurrent episode, Severe
F33.3	Major depressive disorder, Recurrent episode, With psychotic features
F33.41	Major depressive disorder, Recurrent episode, In partial remission
F33.42	Major depressive disorder, Recurrent episode, In full remission
F33.9	Major depressive disorder, Recurrent episode, Unspecified
F34.0	Cyclothymic disorder
F34.1	Persistent depressive disorder
F34.81	Disruptive mood dysregulation disorder
F39	Unspecified mood disorder
F40.00	Agoraphobia
F40.10	Social anxiety disorder
F40.218	Specific phobia, Animal
F40.228	Specific phobia, Natural environment
F40.230	Specific phobia, Fear of blood
F40.231	Specific phobia, Fear of injections and transfusions
F40.232	Specific phobia, Fear of other medical care
F40.233	Specific phobia, Fear of injury
F40.248	Specific phobia, Situational
F40.298	Specific phobia, Other
F41.0	Panic disorder
F41.1	Generalized anxiety disorder

ICD-10-CM Disorder, condition, or problem

F41.8	Other specified anxiety disorder
F41.9	Unspecified anxiety disorder
F42.2	Obsessive-compulsive disorder
F42.3	Hoarding disorder
F42.4	Excoriation (skin-picking) disorder
F42.8	Other specified obsessive-compulsive and related disorder
F42.9	Unspecified obsessive-compulsive and related disorder
F43.0	Acute stress disorder
F43.10	Posttraumatic stress disorder
F43.20	Adjustment disorders, Unspecified
F43.21	Adjustment disorders, With depressed mood
F43.22	Adjustment disorders, With anxiety
F43.23	Adjustment disorders, With mixed anxiety and depressed mood
F43.24	Adjustment disorders, With disturbance of conduct
F43.25	Adjustment disorders, With mixed disturbance of emotions and conduct
F43.81	Prolonged grief disorder
F43.89	Other specified trauma- and stressor-related disorder
F43.9	Unspecified trauma- and stressor-related disorder
F44.0	Dissociative amnesia
F44.1	Dissociative amnesia, With dissociative fugue
F44.4	Functional neurological symptom disorder (conversion disorder), With abnormal movement
F44.4	Functional neurological symptom disorder (conversion disorder), With speech symptom

ICD-10-CM	Disorder, condition, or problem
F44.4	Functional neurological symptom disorder (conversion disorder), With swallowing symptoms
F44.4	Functional neurological symptom disorder (conversion disorder), With weakness/paralysis
F44.5	Functional neurological symptom disorder (conversion disorder), With attacks or seizures
F44.6	Functional neurological symptom disorder (conversion disorder), With anesthesia or sensory loss
F44.6	Functional neurological symptom disorder (conversion disorder), With special sensory symptom
F44.7	Functional neurological symptom disorder (conversion disorder), With mixed symptoms
F44.81	Dissociative identity disorder
F44.89	Other specified dissociative disorder
F44.9	Unspecified dissociative disorder
F45.1	Somatic symptom disorder
F45.21	Illness anxiety disorder
F45.22	Body dysmorphic disorder
F45.8	Other specified somatic symptom and related disorder
F45.9	Unspecified somatic symptom and related disorder
F48.1	Depersonalization/derealization disorder
F50.01	Anorexia nervosa, Restricting type
F50.02	Anorexia nervosa, Binge-eating/purging type
F50.2	Bulimia nervosa
F50.81	Binge-eating disorder
F50.82	Avoidant/restrictive food intake disorder

ICD-10-CM Disorder, condition, or problem

ICD-10-CM	Disorder, condition, or problem
F50.89	Other specified feeding or eating disorder
F50.89	Pica, in adults
F50.9	Unspecified feeding or eating disorder
F51.01	Insomnia disorder
F51.11	Hypersomnolence disorder
F51.3	Non–rapid eye movement sleep arousal disorders, Sleepwalking type
F51.4	Non–rapid eye movement sleep arousal disorders, Sleep terror type
F51.5	Nightmare disorder
F52.0	Male hypoactive sexual desire disorder
F52.21	Erectile disorder
F52.22	Female sexual interest/arousal disorder
F52.31	Female orgasmic disorder
F52.32	Delayed ejaculation
F52.4	Premature (early) ejaculation
F52.6	Genito-pelvic pain/penetration disorder
F52.8	Other specified sexual dysfunction
F52.9	Unspecified sexual dysfunction
F54	Psychological factors affecting other medical conditions
F60.0	Paranoid personality disorder
F60.1	Schizoid personality disorder
F60.2	Antisocial personality disorder
F60.3	Borderline personality disorder
F60.4	Histrionic personality disorder
F60.5	Obsessive-compulsive personality disorder
F60.6	Avoidant personality disorder

ICD-10-CM	Disorder, condition, or problem
F60.7	Dependent personality disorder
F60.81	Narcissistic personality disorder
F60.89	Other specified personality disorder
F60.9	Unspecified personality disorder
F63.0	Gambling disorder
F63.1	Pyromania
F63.2	Kleptomania
F63.3	Trichotillomania (hair-pulling disorder)
F63.81	Intermittent explosive disorder
F64.0	Gender dysphoria in adolescents and adults
F64.2	Gender dysphoria in children
F64.8	Other specified gender dysphoria
F64.9	Unspecified gender dysphoria
F65.0	Fetishistic disorder
F65.1	Transvestic disorder
F65.2	Exhibitionistic disorder
F65.3	Voyeuristic disorder
F65.4	Pedophilic disorder
F65.51	Sexual masochism disorder
F65.52	Sexual sadism disorder
F65.81	Frotteuristic disorder
F65.89	Other specified paraphilic disorder
F65.9	Unspecified paraphilic disorder
F68.10	Factitious disorder imposed on self
F68.A	Factitious disorder imposed on another
F70	Intellectual developmental disorder (intellectual disability), Mild

ICD-10-CM Disorder, condition, or problem

ICD-10-CM	Disorder, condition, or problem
F71	Intellectual developmental disorder (intellectual disability), Moderate
F72	Intellectual developmental disorder (intellectual disability), Severe
F73	Intellectual developmental disorder (intellectual disability), Profound
F79	Unspecified intellectual developmental disorder (intellectual disability)
F80.0	Speech sound disorder
F80.2	Language disorder
F80.81	Childhood-onset fluency disorder (stuttering)
F80.82	Social (pragmatic) communication disorder
F80.9	Unspecified communication disorder
F81.0	Specific learning disorder, With impairment in reading
F81.2	Specific learning disorder, With impairment in mathematics
F81.81	Specific learning disorder, With impairment in written expression
F82	Developmental coordination disorder
F84.0	Autism spectrum disorder
F88	Global developmental delay
F88	Other specified neurodevelopmental disorder
F89	Unspecified neurodevelopmental disorder
F90.0	Attention-deficit/hyperactivity disorder, Predominantly inattentive presentation
F90.1	Attention-deficit/hyperactivity disorder, Predominantly hyperactive/impulsive presentation

ICD-10-CM	Disorder, condition, or problem
F90.2	Attention-deficit/hyperactivity disorder, Combined presentation
F90.8	Other specified attention-deficit/hyperactivity disorder
F90.9	Unspecified attention-deficit/hyperactivity disorder
F91.1	Conduct disorder, Childhood-onset type
F91.2	Conduct disorder, Adolescent-onset type
F91.3	Oppositional defiant disorder
F91.8	Other specified disruptive, impulse-control, and conduct disorder
F91.9	Conduct disorder, Unspecified onset
F91.9	Unspecified disruptive, impulse-control, and conduct disorder
F93.0	Separation anxiety disorder
F94.0	Selective mutism
F94.1	Reactive attachment disorder
F94.2	Disinhibited social engagement disorder
F95.0	Provisional tic disorder
F95.1	Persistent (chronic) motor or vocal tic disorder
F95.2	Tourette's disorder
F95.8	Other specified tic disorder
F95.9	Unspecified tic disorder
F98.0	Enuresis
F98.1	Encopresis
F98.21	Rumination disorder
F98.3	Pica, in children
F98.4	Stereotypic movement disorder
F98.5	Adult-onset fluency disorder

ICD-10-CM   Disorder, condition, or problem

F99	Other specified mental disorder
F99	Unspecified mental disorder
G21.0	Neuroleptic malignant syndrome
G21.11	Antipsychotic medication– and other dopamine receptor blocking agent–induced parkinsonism
G21.19	Other medication-induced parkinsonism
G24.01	Tardive dyskinesia
G24.02	Medication-induced acute dystonia
G24.09	Tardive dystonia
G25.1	Medication-induced postural tremor
G25.71	Medication-induced acute akathisia
G25.71	Tardive akathisia
G25.79	Other medication-induced movement disorder
G25.81	Restless legs syndrome
G31.84	Mild neurocognitive disorder due to possible Alzheimer's disease
G31.84	Mild neurocognitive disorder due to possible frontotemporal degeneration
G31.84	Mild neurocognitive disorder with possible Lewy bodies
G31.84	Mild neurocognitive disorder possibly due to Parkinson's disease
G31.84	Mild neurocognitive disorder possibly due to vascular disease
G31.84	Mild neurocognitive disorder due to unknown etiology
G47.00	Unspecified insomnia disorder
G47.09	Other specified insomnia disorder
G47.10	Unspecified hypersomnolence disorder

ICD-10-CM	Disorder, condition, or problem
G47.19	Other specified hypersomnolence disorder
G47.20	Circadian rhythm sleep-wake disorders, Unspecified type
G47.21	Circadian rhythm sleep-wake disorders, Delayed sleep phase type
G47.22	Circadian rhythm sleep-wake disorders, Advanced sleep phase type
G47.23	Circadian rhythm sleep-wake disorders, Irregular sleep-wake type
G47.24	Circadian rhythm sleep-wake disorders, Non-24-hour sleep-wake type
G47.26	Circadian rhythm sleep-wake disorders, Shift work type
G47.31	Central sleep apnea, Idiopathic central sleep apnea
G47.33	Obstructive sleep apnea hypopnea
G47.34	Sleep-related hypoventilation, Idiopathic hypoventilation
G47.35	Sleep-related hypoventilation, Congenital central alveolar hypoventilation
G47.36	Sleep-related hypoventilation, Comorbid sleep-related hypoventilation
G47.37	Central sleep apnea comorbid with opioid use
G47.411	Narcolepsy with cataplexy or hypocretin deficiency (type 1)
G47.419	Narcolepsy without cataplexy and either without hypocretin deficiency or hypocretin unmeasured (type 2)
G47.421	Narcolepsy with cataplexy or hypocretin deficiency due to a medical condition
G47.429	Narcolepsy without cataplexy and without hypocretin deficiency due to a medical condition

ICD-10-CM Disorder, condition, or problem

G47.52	Rapid eye movement sleep behavior disorder
G47.8	Other specified sleep-wake disorder
G47.9	Unspecified sleep-wake disorder
N39.498	Other specified elimination disorder, With urinary symptoms
R06.3	Central sleep apnea, Cheyne-Stokes breathing
R15.9	Other specified elimination disorder, With fecal symptoms
R15.9	Unspecified elimination disorder, With fecal symptoms
R32	Unspecified elimination disorder, With urinary symptoms
R41.81	Age-related cognitive decline
R41.83	Borderline intellectual functioning
R41.9	Unspecified neurocognitive disorder
R45.88	Current nonsuicidal self-injury
R45.89	Impairing emotional outbursts
T14.91XA	Current suicidal behavior, Initial encounter
T14.91XD	Current suicidal behavior, Subsequent encounter
T43.205A	Antidepressant discontinuation syndrome, Initial encounter
T43.205D	Antidepressant discontinuation syndrome, Subsequent encounter
T43.205S	Antidepressant discontinuation syndrome, Sequelae
T50.905A	Other adverse effect of medication, Initial encounter
T50.905D	Other adverse effect of medication, Subsequent encounter
T50.905S	Other adverse effect of medication, Sequelae

ICD-10-CM	Disorder, condition, or problem
T74.01XA	Spouse or partner neglect, Confirmed, Initial encounter
T74.01XD	Spouse or partner neglect, Confirmed, Subsequent encounter
T74.02XA	Child neglect, Confirmed, Initial encounter
T74.02XD	Child neglect, Confirmed, Subsequent encounter
T74.11XA	Adult physical abuse by nonspouse or nonpartner, Confirmed, Initial encounter
T74.11XA	Spouse or partner violence, Physical, Confirmed, Initial encounter
T74.11XD	Adult physical abuse by nonspouse or nonpartner, Confirmed, Subsequent encounter
T74.11XD	Spouse or partner violence, Physical, Confirmed, Subsequent encounter
T74.12XA	Child physical abuse, Confirmed, Initial encounter
T74.12XD	Child physical abuse, Confirmed, Subsequent encounter
T74.21XA	Adult sexual abuse by nonspouse or nonpartner, Confirmed, Initial encounter
T74.21XA	Spouse or partner violence, Sexual, Confirmed, Initial encounter
T74.21XD	Adult sexual abuse by nonspouse or nonpartner, Confirmed, Subsequent encounter
T74.21XD	Spouse or partner violence, Sexual, Confirmed, Subsequent encounter
T74.22XA	Child sexual abuse, Confirmed, Initial encounter
T74.22XD	Child sexual abuse, Confirmed, Subsequent encounter
T74.31XA	Adult psychological abuse by nonspouse or nonpartner, Confirmed, Initial encounter

ICD-10-CM	Disorder, condition, or problem
T74.31XA	Spouse or partner abuse, Psychological, Confirmed, Initial encounter
T74.31XD	Adult psychological abuse by nonspouse or nonpartner, Confirmed, Subsequent encounter
T74.31XD	Spouse or partner abuse, Psychological, Confirmed, Subsequent encounter
T74.32XA	Child psychological abuse, Confirmed, Initial encounter
T74.32XD	Child psychological abuse, Confirmed, Subsequent encounter
T76.01XA	Spouse or partner neglect, Suspected, Initial encounter
T76.01XD	Spouse or partner neglect, Suspected, Subsequent encounter
T76.02XA	Child neglect, Suspected, Initial encounter
T76.02XD	Child neglect, Suspected, Subsequent encounter
T76.11XA	Adult physical abuse by nonspouse or nonpartner, Suspected, Initial encounter
T76.11XA	Spouse or partner violence, Physical, Suspected, Initial encounter
T76.11XD	Adult physical abuse by nonspouse or nonpartner, Suspected, Subsequent encounter
T76.11XD	Spouse or partner violence, Physical, Suspected, Subsequent encounter
T76.12XA	Child physical abuse, Suspected, Initial encounter
T76.12XD	Child physical abuse, Suspected, Subsequent encounter
T76.21XA	Adult sexual abuse by nonspouse or nonpartner, Suspected, Initial encounter
T76.21XA	Spouse or partner violence, Sexual, Suspected, Initial encounter

ICD-10-CM Disorder, condition, or problem

T76.21XD	Adult sexual abuse by nonspouse or nonpartner, Suspected, Subsequent encounter
T76.21XD	Spouse or partner violence, Sexual, Suspected, Subsequent encounter
T76.22XA	Child sexual abuse, Suspected, Initial encounter
T76.22XD	Child sexual abuse, Suspected, Subsequent encounter
T76.31XA	Adult psychological abuse by nonspouse or nonpartner, Suspected, Initial encounter
T76.31XA	Spouse or partner abuse, Psychological, Suspected, Initial encounter
T76.31XD	Adult psychological abuse by nonspouse or nonpartner, Suspected, Subsequent encounter
T76.31XD	Spouse or partner abuse, Psychological, Suspected, Subsequent encounter
T76.32XA	Child psychological abuse, Suspected, Initial encounter
T76.32XD	Child psychological abuse, Suspected, Subsequent encounter
Z03.89	No diagnosis or condition
Z31.5	Genetic counseling
Z55.0	Illiteracy and low-level literacy
Z55.1	Schooling unavailable and unattainable
Z55.2	Failed school examinations
Z55.3	Underachievement in school
Z55.4	Educational maladjustment and discord with teachers and classmates
Z55.8	Problems related to inadequate teaching
Z55.9	Other problems related to education and literacy
Z56.0	Unemployment

ICD-10-CM   Disorder, condition, or problem

Z56.1	Change of job
Z56.2	Threat of job loss
Z56.3	Stressful work schedule
Z56.4	Discord with boss and workmates
Z56.5	Uncongenial work environment
Z56.6	Other physical and mental strain related to work
Z56.81	Sexual harassment on the job
Z56.82	Problem related to current military deployment status
Z56.9	Other problem related to employment
Z58.6	Lack of safe drinking water
Z59.01	Sheltered homelessness
Z59.02	Unsheltered homelessness
Z59.10	Inadequate housing
Z59.2	Discord with neighbor, lodger, or landlord
Z59.3	Problem related to living in a residential institution
Z59.41	Food insecurity
Z59.5	Extreme poverty
Z59.6	Low income
Z59.7	Insufficient social or health insurance or welfare support
Z59.9	Other economic problem
Z59.9	Other housing problem
Z60.0	Phase of life problem
Z60.2	Problem related to living alone
Z60.3	Acculturation difficulty
Z60.4	Social exclusion or rejection
Z60.5	Target of (perceived) adverse discrimination or persecution

ICD-10-CM	Disorder, condition, or problem
Z60.9	Other problem related to social environment
Z62.29	Upbringing away from parents
Z62.810	Personal history (past history) of physical abuse in childhood
Z62.810	Personal history (past history) of sexual abuse in childhood
Z62.811	Personal history (past history) of psychological abuse in childhood
Z62.812	Personal history (past history) of neglect in childhood
Z62.820	Parent-child relational problem, Parent–biological child
Z62.821	Parent-child relational problem, Parent–adopted child
Z62.822	Parent-child relational problem, Parent–foster child
Z62.891	Sibling relational problem
Z62.898	Child affected by parental relationship distress
Z62.898	Parent-child relational problem, Other caregiver–child
Z63.0	Relationship distress with spouse or intimate partner
Z63.4	Uncomplicated bereavement
Z63.5	Disruption of family by separation or divorce
Z63.8	High expressed emotion level within family
Z64.0	Problems related to unwanted pregnancy
Z64.1	Problems related to multiparity
Z64.4	Discord with social service provider, including probation officer, case manager, or social services worker
Z65.0	Conviction in civil or criminal proceedings without imprisonment
Z65.1	Imprisonment or other incarceration

ICD-10-CM Disorder, condition, or problem

Z65.2	Problems related to release from prison
Z65.3	Problems related to other legal circumstances
Z65.4	Victim of crime
Z65.4	Victim of terrorism or torture
Z65.5	Exposure to disaster, war, or other hostilities
Z65.8	Religious or spiritual problem
Z69.010	Encounter for mental health services for victim of child neglect by parent
Z69.010	Encounter for mental health services for victim of child physical abuse by parent
Z69.010	Encounter for mental health services for victim of child psychological abuse by parent
Z69.010	Encounter for mental health services for victim of child sexual abuse by parent
Z69.011	Encounter for mental health services for perpetrator of parental child neglect
Z69.011	Encounter for mental health services for perpetrator of parental child physical abuse
Z69.011	Encounter for mental health services for perpetrator of parental child psychological abuse
Z69.011	Encounter for mental health services for perpetrator of parental child sexual abuse
Z69.020	Encounter for mental health services for victim of nonparental child neglect
Z69.020	Encounter for mental health services for victim of nonparental child physical abuse
Z69.020	Encounter for mental health services for victim of nonparental child psychological abuse
Z69.020	Encounter for mental health services for victim of nonparental child sexual abuse

ICD-10-CM	Disorder, condition, or problem
Z69.021	Encounter for mental health services for perpetrator of nonparental child neglect
Z69.021	Encounter for mental health services for perpetrator of nonparental child physical abuse
Z69.021	Encounter for mental health services for perpetrator of nonparental child psychological abuse
Z69.021	Encounter for mental health services for perpetrator of nonparental child sexual abuse
Z69.11	Encounter for mental health services for victim of spouse or partner neglect
Z69.11	Encounter for mental health services for victim of spouse or partner psychological abuse
Z69.11	Encounter for mental health services for victim of spouse or partner violence, Physical
Z69.12	Encounter for mental health services for perpetrator of spouse or partner neglect
Z69.12	Encounter for mental health services for perpetrator of spouse or partner psychological abuse
Z69.12	Encounter for mental health services for perpetrator of spouse or partner violence, Physical
Z69.12	Encounter for mental health services for perpetrator of spouse or partner violence, Sexual
Z69.81	Encounter for mental health services for victim of nonspousal or nonpartner adult abuse
Z69.81	Encounter for mental health services for victim of spouse or partner violence, Sexual
Z69.82	Encounter for mental health services for perpetrator of nonspousal or nonpartner adult abuse
Z70.9	Sex counseling
Z71.3	Dietary counseling
Z71.9	Other counseling or consultation

ICD-10-CM	Disorder, condition, or problem
Z72.0	Tobacco use disorder, mild
Z72.810	Child or adolescent antisocial behavior
Z72.811	Adult antisocial behavior
Z72.9	Problem related to lifestyle
Z75.3	Unavailability or inaccessibility of health care facilities
Z75.4	Unavailability or inaccessibility of other helping agencies
Z76.5	Malingering
Z91.199	Nonadherence to medical treatment
Z91.410	Personal history (past history) of spouse or partner violence, Physical
Z91.410	Personal history (past history) of spouse or partner violence, Sexual
Z91.411	Personal history (past history) of spouse or partner psychological abuse
Z91.412	Personal history (past history) of spouse or partner neglect
Z91.49	Personal history of psychological trauma
Z91.51	History of suicidal behavior
Z91.52	History of nonsuicidal self-injury
Z91.82	Personal history of military deployment
Z91.83	Wandering associated with a mental disorder